IMMERSE YOURSELF
IN THE LUSCIOUS TASTES
OF THE MEDITERRANEAN . . .

Thick, dark bread full of whole grains . . .

The freshest vegetables—wild greens, zucchini, spinach, peas, tomatoes, and mushrooms

Whole grains including risotto and pilaf; pasta from Italian spaghetti to Moroccan couscous and polenta . . .

Protein-rich legumes such as lentils, chickpeas, fava beans, white haricot beans, and cranberry beans . . .

Succulent fruits like peaches, cantaloupe, watermelon, figs, and grapes

Flavorings from garlic, onion, and lemon to basil, oregano, parsley, cilantro, and olive oil . . .

"Beyond the ingredients themselves, eating the traditional Mediterranean way is a philosophy in itself: Life is for savoring, and food is a glorious and beautiful expression of life. Meals are gathering of family and friends, genuine events, not inconvenient chores. Food sustains life."

—from *The Mediterranean Diet*

THE
MEDITERRANEAN
DIET

Marissa Cloutier, MS, RD
and Eve Adamson

Produced by Amaranth

HarperTorch
An Imprint of HarperCollinsPublishers

THE MEDITERRANEAN DIET is not a substitute for sound medical advice. The ideas, procedures, and suggestions in this book are intended to supplement, not replace, the medical advice of a trained medical professional. All matters regarding your health require medical supervision. Consult your physician before adopting any suggestions in this book, as well as about any condition that may require diagnosis or medical attention. The authors, publisher, and book producer disclaim any liability arising directly or indirectly from the use of this book.

HARPERTORCH
An Imprint of HarperCollins*Publishers*
10 East 53rd Street
New York, New York 10022-5299

Copyright © 2001 by Amaranth
ISBN: 0-380-81441-2

First HarperTorch paperback printing: January 2001

HarperCollins®, HarperTorch™, and ◆™ are trademarks of Harper-Collins Publishers Inc.

Printed in the United States of America

Visit HarperTorch on the World Wide Web at www.harpercollins.com

10 9 8 7 6 5 4 3 2

This book is dedicated to my mother,
Merna Lattimer,
and my grandmother,
Letita Del Prete-Asta.
Bona salute, Lunga vit.
(Good health, Long life)
—M. C.

To my children, Angus and Emmett,
that they may learn to eat well, live well,
and take their health into their own hands.
—E. A.

Acknowledgments

I would like to thank Normand J. Cloutier, Ph.D.; Michael D. Cloutier; Gail Zyla, M.S., R.D.; Mary Thang; and Sharon Lee Asta for their support and inspiration.

—M. C.

Thanks to my parents, my most appreciative taste testers for the past fifteen years.

—E. A.

Contents

Introduction

If you grew up with a television set, you've probably seen the familiar scenario: a family gathered around the breakfast table, their plates piled high with eggs, bacon, sausage, maybe even a breakfast steak, and a formidable stack of pancakes. A bottle of maple-flavored syrup and a stick of butter (or tub of margarine) were fixtures at the center of the table. A large glass of whole milk and a small glass of orange juice stood sentinel in front of every plate. A mother, coiffed and smiling, urged the family to finish the "nutritious" breakfast, that "most important meal of the day!"

One has to wonder how Americans got the idea that steak and eggs for breakfast made for a healthy meal. And what about dinner? America's "ideal" dinner in the 1950s and 1960s consisted of a large hunk of meat and a baked potato with butter and sour cream, along with a stack of white bread and butter and possibly a small bowl of iceberg lettuce and a few carrot shreds on the side or a few spoonfuls of overcooked, heavily salted, buttered vegetables. We all thought this sort of "home cooking" made us strong and healthy, didn't we? Not to mention, we got pretty accustomed to that comfort-food taste.

So why on earth would we want to switch to unadorned,

whole-grain cereal and fruit for breakfast, or salads and vegetable soups for dinner, with (the horror!) no cream and butter to help them go down? Why would we want to eat whole-grain bread when the neat white stuff is so cheap and readily available? And why would we give up that big dish of ice cream, slab of cake, or wedge of apple pie à la mode for dessert in favor of a bowl of fruit?

Then again, why would we want to eat in a manner that has made America one of the leading countries in the number of heart attacks per year? Surely Mom's home cooking isn't killing us off—or is it?

The irony of the situation is that while 1950s Americans were happily downing forkfuls of high-fat fare in enjoyment of their prosperity, at the same time in history, the people living around the Mediterranean Sea, in regions less wealthy and with food budgets far lower, were eating what scientists and researchers have recently discovered is one of the healthiest ways to eat in the world. Today, as Americans struggle to retain or regain their coronary health, they are turning to the latest, cutting-edge research for guidance, and that research is pointing with increased frequency toward the traditional cuisines of the working class in the Mediterranean region as seen during the 1950s and 1960s and before. Sometimes, progress means looking backward—and, in this case, to another continent.

The problem is, Americans love their food, and aren't quick to adopt any program, guideline, or advice that takes them away from their beloved burgers and fries. This fact alone makes the traditional Mediterranean diet worth a second—and third, and daily—look. What is so special about the traditional Mediterranean diet? Why, for the past forty years or so, have researchers been excited about the traditional dietary habits of the people around the Mediterranean Sea? Aren't eating habits from so many years ago outmoded today, when so many cutting-edge food products line our supermarket shelves? Isn't progress the name of the game? Those frozen dinners don't taste too bad . . .

First, let's look at how Americans have developed their ideas about nutrition and what makes for a healthy meal. Without an understanding of how our own preconceptions developed, a change in diet probably won't be effective. Why do we eat what we eat? And how do we know what to eat now? What does the research say?

✥ THE GOLDEN AGE OF NUTRITION

In the early part of the twentieth century, nutrition science was in its infancy but growing fast. Many exciting and significant advances in nutritional knowledge were made between 1910 and 1960, particularly the discovery of specific nutrients and their biochemical relationship to human health. What was required to maintain health and support growth and reproduction? And what would happen when certain nutrients were missing? These were the questions that concerned nutrition scientists of the day.

During this period, scientists learned that without vitamin C, people develop scurvy, without vitamin A, night blindness. Vitamin D deficiencies lead to rickets in children, thiamin deficiencies to beriberi, niacin deficiencies to pellagra, and calcium deficiencies to stunted growth in children and osteoporosis later in life. Iron deficiencies lead to anemia, iodine deficiencies to goiter, and zinc deficiencies to growth failure in children. These conditions are classics in nutrition science today, and have all led to an understanding that a certain nutrient profile is necessary for health. The emphasis of research was on what might be missing from our diets that could compromise our health.

One significant example of this research emphasis was in the work of several British investigators, including Corey Mann and Boyd Orr, who attempted to remedy the problem of why the working classes in northern England and Scotland—the groups reproducing at a higher rate than the aristocracy—seemed to be getting shorter and thinner. The government of Great Britain was concerned. The notion that the "lower" classes were simply genetically inferior was a prominent one, but how could Britain compete in an increasingly global world as a colonial power if their very genetic stock was degenerating? Was there anything they could do to restore the working class? Was the answer within the realm of human control?

Mann and Orr embarked upon an investigation to determine whether anything could be done to induce growth in short children. Sure enough, the results of feeding studies using short children as subjects revealed that feeding butter and sugar induced weight gain but no height increase; children fed milk or meat supplements, on the other hand, grew taller. The British working class wasn't genetically lacking—it was malnourished! Public policy began to evolve in conjunction with farmers and social activists to provide milk in schools, milk and orange juice to pregnant and nursing mothers, and, once the war began, milk and meat rations equally to all classes. Food production became a major priority for many nations, not just Great Britain. "Avoid deficiencies" was the battle cry.

Once World War II hit and the possibility arose that the "enemy" might be able to prohibit the importation of food, food production and rationing took on an even greater importance. Agricultural policy shifted to emphasize the production of milk and meat to ensure the welfare of children, the "nation's future." Agricultural autonomy became a matter of national survival as well as national pride.

❧ POSTWAR NUTRITIONAL PRIORITIES

Since the war, efficient food production has been the order of the day for developed countries all over the world. Science applied to farming methods in the form of pesticides, fertilizers, growth regulators, and genetic selection has resulted in higher yields from crops, more efficient production of livestock and dairy herds, and agricultural policies that distinguish farmers from all other business industries. Farming became big business—ultraefficient and a major moneymaker, too.

The second major development since the war was in the area of food processing. Processed food—in cans, in dried form, and otherwise packaged for our convenience—is a relatively new phenomenon. Packaged food, often enriched, seemed to be a cheap and efficient way to feed the masses. Because the current climate emphasized the need for calories and the inclusion of all the required micronutrients (to prevent stunted growth, for example, or a range of other health problems), the food industry's invention and production of ready-made foods seemed to represent a revolution in nutrition. As long as these products had sufficient calories and micronutrients, little thought was given to what else they might contain: high fat and sugar content, preservatives, highly refined ingredients, and so on. These products were easily distributed, lasted a long time, and seemed to represent an efficient way to meet the energy requirements of a large population. Most nutritionists of the day were in favor of this new trend.

Even today, the notion that deficiency prevention should be the primary nutritional objective exists in the minds and policies of politicians, physicians, and the food industry. Of course, preventing nutritional deficiencies is still important. If micronutrients are lacking in the diet, health problems will still occur. However, the previous approach, which emphasized sufficient calories and micronutrient deficiency prevention, has led to problems the policymakers before World War II could hardly have foreseen. Our technologically advanced and vastly automated society has a lower need for calories, or energy, than it once did in a more labor-intensive climate. (Even farming, once a very hard and active lifestyle, has, on the whole, become largely machine-driven.) Less physical activity translates to fewer calorie needs. Also, we are discovering that highly processed and packaged food sometimes contains additional undesirable elements—too many calories, too much sugar, too much fat, for example—and may also lack components such as phytochemicals and fiber not previously factored into nutritional requirements.

ℬ THE MEDITERRANEAN DIET: BEYOND ADEQUATE

But what does all this have to do with the Mediterranean diet? As America and Great Britain shifted their focus toward meat and milk as well as toward the efficient feeding of large numbers of people, those living in the Mediterranean region after World War II continued to eat much the way they had eaten for centuries, their diet peacefully undiscovered. With diets consisting primarily of plant foods instead of foods from animal sources, people in the Mediterranean region were enjoying exceptionally low levels of coronary heart disease and other chronic diseases, such as certain forms of cancer.

The first major study to examine the diet of people living in the Mediterranean was a comprehensive and astonishingly thorough examination of the diets of the people living on the island of Crete in 1948. The Greek government, in an attempt to improve the postwar conditions of its country, turned to the industrialized nations for advice. In response, the Rockefeller Foundation assigned epidemiologist Leland Allbaugh to the case.

Whether or not everyone assumed the animal protein–based diet of the industrialized nations would be superior to the plant-based diet of underdeveloped Crete, the results of the Rockefeller Foundation study were surprising. Far from presenting a bleak health picture of poverty, malnourishment, starvation, and ill health, the Cretan diet, according to the foundation researchers, was "surprisingly good." Deriving approximately 61 percent of its calories from plant foods, only 7 percent from animal foods, and a full 38 percent of total calories from fat (similar to the percentage of fat in the United States food supply of the late 1940s, but primarily from olive oil and olives rather than from animal fats), the diet was indeed more than "surprisingly good." It was very conducive to health, specifically heart health.

Ironically, however, Allbaugh's final analysis included a recommendation that the Cretan diet could be improved with more foods of animal origin, primarily because study respondents generally expressed a wish for more meat, rice, fish, pasta, butter, and cheese (in that order) in their diets. A full 72 percent of people in the survey named meat as their favorite food. In contemporary

Crete, foods of animal origin make up a greater percentage of the diet than they once did. One recent study of the urban population of Crete found increased intake of animal products and a decreased intake of bread, fruit, potatoes, and olive oil compared to the 1960s diet. Similar changes in other Mediterranean countries are also evident, and scientists have also observed an increase in the rate of coronary heart disease, diabetes, and several types of cancers in the Mediterranean region today.

The Rockefeller Foundation study was the first major study to examine the diets of those living in the Mediterranean. Since then, researchers have studied why people living in these areas were living longer lives and enjoying far lower rates of coronary heart disease and other chronic diseases. Study after study examining the traditional diets of the Mediterranean region has supported the notion that a primarily plant-based diet may indeed be at the heart of longer life and better health.

ℬ RECENT TRENDS

The message is still prevalent in the minds of people living in the Western world: eat animal protein and lots of it. One unfortunate result of this dictum has been an overemphasis on foods that contain a high amount of saturated fat. This also results in a de-emphasis on plant foods, which scientists are discovering contain a wide array of health-promoting compounds such as fiber, antioxidants, and phytochemicals.

As public health issues change and nutritional science advances, it pays to be aware of a few past misconceptions. People tend to overlook the fact that the studies advocating the feeding of animal protein supplements were conducted on children whose growth was stunted due to malnutrition. Milk and meat are certainly beneficial in the diets of children. For full-grown adults, milk (especially low fat or nonfat) can support the maintenance of bone structure. However, in general, the average, healthy adult American (not including pregnant or breast-feeding mothers, or others with special nutritional needs) tends to consume far above the baseline protein need.

The link between saturated-fat consumption and heart disease has not gone unnoticed. Around 1970, the beef industry and the dairy industry both began to produce lower-fat products. The word in the media was that fat was bad—saturated fat in particular, but in general, all fat. Other food-industry sectors responded, as well. Hundreds of low-fat and nonfat versions of our favorite foods appeared on supermarket shelves and were purchased with enthusiasm. The Mediterranean diet, already proclaimed by the media as a healthful alternative to the standard American diet, became known as just another low–saturated fat eating plan.

In the early 1990s, research further illuminated the differences between types of fats. Scientists Frank Sacks and Walter Willett, among others, recognized that high levels of a certain type of blood cholesterol—HDL, or what has become known as "good cholesterol"—could actually be just as important for coronary heart disease prevention as low levels of total blood cholesterol, or of "bad" (LDL) blood cholesterol. Because diets low in saturated fats and high in monounsaturated fats appear to increase HDL cholesterol in addition to lowering LDL cholesterol, the Mediterranean diet again became a topic of interest. Olive oil, the principal fat in the Mediterranean diet, is a rich source of monounsaturated fat. This, surmised scientists, could be an important contributor to the lower levels of coronary heart disease in the Mediterranean region.

In addition, research began to reveal that hydrogenated vegetable fats, such as those used to create margarine and vegetable shortening, may actually contribute to heart disease risk. Fat in the diet was no longer simply a matter of percentage. Fat in the Mediterranean diet, researchers began to realize, was distinctly different from fat in the standard American diet, even if the percentages of total calories from fat were similar.

✀ THE FUTURE OF NUTRITION

As nutrition science evolves, consumers and scientists alike may still find it difficult to get past this basic mantra of deficiency prevention. Once again, deficiency prevention is an essential part of a complete nutritional profile. Many of the "traditional" vitamins and minerals scientists have known about for many decades remain an important part of the fight against heart disease and cancer, especially vitamin E, folacin, and selenium. The Mediterranean diet, with its emphasis on vegetables, fruit, and whole grains, is an excellent and complete diet that will not result in nutrient deficiencies and is compatible with excellent health.

However, a new movement is taking place in the area of nutrition. This new way of thinking, called the "second Golden Age of Nutrition" by Mark Messina, Ph.D., a soy foods expert and former researcher with the National Cancer Institute's Diet and Cancer Branch, concerns itself with what we include in our diets—specifically, the wide array of compounds in plant foods called phytochemicals—rather than what is missing.

Phytochemicals are chemical compounds in plants.

These include the well-known vitamins C and E and the oft-touted beta-carotene. They also include thousands of other nutrients not formerly a part of the layman's nutrition vocabulary: lycopene, the substance that makes tomatoes and red peppers red, and allium, the compound that gives garlic its unique aroma, just to name a few.

The latest research into phytochemicals is promising, and according to scientists studying phytochemicals, these plant compounds may support our health in more ways than we can imagine, from slowing the aging process and strengthening our immune systems against disease to preventing or even reversing chronic conditions such as cancer and heart disease.

The traditional Mediterranean diet's emphasis on plant foods (including olive oil) makes it a rich source of phytochemicals, as well as HDL-boosting monounsaturated fats. Truly a diet for the new millennium, the traditional Mediterranean diet is the best of paradoxes: an ancient eating tradition with cutting-edge health benefits that is both simple to prepare and indescribably delicious (not that we won't try our best to describe it!).

And so we come to the purpose of this book: to explore the traditional Mediterranean diet in terms of how it can improve the health, well-being, longevity, and quality of life for those of us living half a century later and thousands of miles away. How can we adjust our own diets, lifestyles, activity levels, even attitudes, for better health, à la the Mediterranean? Can we improve on the traditional Mediterranean diet to make it more compatible with our contemporary lifestyles and preferences? Is creating health for ourselves as simple as indulging in simple, fragrant, gratifying meals? These are the questions this book will address. We hope you will join us on our sun-drenched, cypress-lined, color-soaked, flavor-rich, and irresistibly delicious journey through the Mediterranean in search of greater longevity, healthier hearts, and a better quality of life. It is sure to be a magnificent vacation, and one that can last all year round. Bon voyage, steak and potatoes! Shall we set sail?

1: *Mediterranean Magic*

Imagine yourself sitting in a sun-drenched outdoor café on the banks of the Greek Mediterranean shore. The vast turquoise sea meets the brilliant blue sky, and everything around you seems influenced by sea and sky, from the aquamarine-painted tables and chairs of the café to the foamy-white buildings and small shops jutting out over the seawall where the Mediterranean laps and splashes. The warm sun on your shoulders and the cool sea breeze on your face enhance the spectacular view, as the fragrance of white flowers scaling a peach-colored trellis above your table mingles with the smells of salt and sea.

You feel yourself relaxing into your chair as you are gently serenaded by the musical dialect around you. You recall your morning trek across the vast white beaches, and images of ancient Greece envelop you. You can almost envision Socrates walking along the shoreline with tall Greek ships sailing in the far distance, the ruins whole, the early blossoming of Western civilization. Poseidon, that great god of the sea, is smiling at you, amused to see how easily the stresses of daily life have suddenly melted away.

Ah, the magical Mediterranean. With all its glorious

old-worldliness, you feel connected with history. You feel completely at peace. And just when you think it couldn't get any better, you are awakened from your relaxed bliss by a waiter who brings you a bowl of fragrant, lemony soup the color of the sun, followed by a steaming plate of sea bass infused with oregano, olive oil, and lemon, surrounded by colorful roasted vegetables grown on the rolling hills just behind you.

With each bite you are catapulted further into the heaven that surrounds you. You cannot help but savor every mouthful. You've never tasted food so fresh, so wholesome. You feel renewed, even healed, down to your very soul.

Indeed, the sensual power of the Mediterranean cannot be ignored. Anyone who has traveled to this area cannot forget its beauty, its history, and its charm. Sun and sea, relaxed lifestyle, and miraculous food. These things are enough to draw anyone to the shores of the Mediterranean. Yet, the seductive Mediterranean climate, cuisine, and way of life aren't the only reasons to focus on this region's approach to eating. Study after study has revealed that people eating a traditional Mediterranean diet are generally healthier, longer-lived, and with a lower incidence of chronic diseases—particularly coronary artery disease—than people in other parts of the world.

The potential health benefits inherent in eating and living in the traditional Mediterranean way are the impetus for writing this book. Is it really possible to eat so well, savoring and relishing delicious food, and at the same time increase our wellness? In fact, it is possible, and also surprisingly easy to accomplish. We need only look to the Mediterranean lands of Greece, Italy, France, Spain, Turkey, North Africa, and the Middle East.

✎ THE MEDITERRANEAN REGION

The Mediterranean region encompasses all the countries bordering the Mediterranean Sea, from the Strait of Gibraltar separating the rocky cliffs and crags of southern Spain and the seaport of Tangier in mountainous northern Morocco, to the Mediterranean's far western reaches along the shores of the Middle East. Between these extremes lies a broad sampling of European, Middle Eastern, and African countries, all Mediterranean yet each unique in culture and character: pastoral southern France with its orange groves, vineyards, and rolling hills; scenic Italy with its snowy peaks and sultry beaches; the former Yugoslavia with its dramatic coastline; the tiny yet sensationally mountainous Albania; historical Greece with its hazy, sea-infused ambience and its scattering of islands; geologically volatile Turkey; the Middle Eastern countries of Syria, Lebanon, and Israel, with their coastal planes backed by a sudden rise of mountains; and then, returning east, the northern ends of Egypt, Libya, Tunisia, Algeria, and back to Morocco, an African panoply of cliffs, peaks, ports, plateaus, and scorching sands.

Surely such a vast array of countries and cultures must dine on an equally vast assortment of foods. Although each country bordering the Mediterranean Sea does indeed have its unique culinary characteristics, the region maintains many common, and many more mutually influenced ingredients, recipes, and cooking techniques. Pasta may come in the form of ziti in Italy and couscous in Morocco, but it is still pasta. Not insignificantly, Mediterranean countries also share an attitude toward food and how it should be eaten.

✎ THE EVOLUTION OF A SHARED CUISINE

The magnificent diet of the Mediterranean region has been evolving for thousands of years. The history of the region coupled with its distinct (though widely various) climate and the pervasive influence of the sea has shaped the choice of foods and the types of cooking so characteristic of traditional Mediterranean culture. Bread, olive oil, and wine—which continue to play a significant role in the Mediterranean diet today—accompanied meals in ancient times. The cultivated vegetables and other plant-based foods so central to the diet can be traced back to Neolithic times. According to archeological evidence and depictions and descriptions of food and meals in the art and literature of ancient Greek and Roman civilizations, ancient populations probably relied primarily on plant foods, with only occasional indulgence in meat and seafood.

More recent studies of the Mediterranean diet, from the 1950s and 1960s, reveal eating habits and preferences similar to the ancient diet: a primarily plant food–based diet that included minimal processing, whole grains, olive oil as the primary fat source, and animal products (with the exception of cheese in some areas and yogurt in some areas) consumed only a few times per month. The groundbreaking Rockefeller Foundation study of the Cretan diet around 1950 stated that "olives, cereal grains, pulses, wild greens and herbs, and fruits, together with limited quantities of goat meat and milk, game, and fish have remained the basic Cretan foods for forty centuries . . . no meal was complete without bread . . . [and] Olives and olive oil contributed heavily to the energy intake." This study, originally undertaken to determine how the people of Greece could improve their diets after

World War II, concluded that the diet couldn't get much better.

While the Mediterranean diet today has strayed from its original roots somewhat (due to the "McDonald's invasion" and other nutritionally tragic "modern" influences, such as the growing popularity of heavily preserved convenience foods), the Mediterranean diet in the first half of the twentieth century, with appropriate modifications to make it more suitable and convenient for contemporary eating, will be the focus of this book.

✤ TO EAT À LA MEDITERRANEAN

Let's look more closely at this traditional diet and its various common components. Eating the traditional Mediterranean way is largely a seasonal and regional affair. While each country has its unique customs, foods produced locally or regionally and served soon after harvest are ubiquitous. In spring, the freshest new vegetables are harvested and eaten, often within a few miles of where they were picked—wild greens, thin zucchini, green beans, spinach, spring peas, finocchi, cherries, and wild mushrooms. Summer marks the arrival of an abundance of tomatoes, eggplant, peaches, cantaloupe, watermelon, figs, peppers, and onions. Outdoor markets offer the freshest fruits and vegetables. The pale, bland produce often available in American supermarkets would be virtually unrecognizable next to the vibrantly colored and succulent array of regionally produced plant foods. Fresh fruit is the most common dessert, and certain vegetables and herbs feature prominently in the cuisines of most Mediterranean countries—most notably, garlic, onions, and tomatoes.

At the end of the summer, the grape harvest and wine

pressing begin. Persimmons and pomegranates follow, and then olives are harvested and pressed to yield the oil so essential to Mediterranean cuisine—and, as we'll discuss later, an important component of the heart-healthy, traditional Mediterranean diet.

Beyond the magnificent year-round harvest of fruits and vegetables and the reliance on olive oil as the principal source of fat, the Mediterranean people shared other dietary similarities. Meat was more luxury than staple, and although many Mediterranean dishes are flavored with meat, those that feature it are usually reserved for special occasions. Lamb and veal are more common than beef because grazing land is scarce in the Mediterranean, and chicken or seafood are more likely to feature prominently in main courses when meat is featured at all.

Bread is a staple, even in Italy, where pasta is consumed so readily. Traditional Mediterranean bread, especially in rural areas, is dark, heavy (some loaves could weigh almost five pounds!), and full of whole grains, unlike the soft, refined white bread neatly sliced and conveniently bagged for American consumers. Whole grains are consumed in abundance outside the obligatory loaf of bread—rice in the form of paella, risotto, and pilaf; pasta in its many incarnations, from Italian spaghetti to Moroccan couscous; and the versatile cornmeal mixture called polenta are favorites. Legumes are another staple—inexpensive and high in protein, they were an essential part of the traditional Mediterranean diet. White haricot beans, small red cranberry beans, lentils, chickpeas, and fava beans remain popular options today.

Another common Mediterranean theme is wine, although it was traditionally consumed primarily by men and always with meals, never recreationally. A small piece of cheese to begin or end a meal was common, but food was never smothered in cheese the way it sometimes is in Americanized Italian dishes. Many Mediterranean dishes share a similar flavor and character due to a few popular flavoring ingredients: garlic, onion, lemons, olive oil, basil, oregano, parsley, Italian parsley, and often a few small pieces of pancetta, an unsmoked bacon.

Beyond the ingredients themselves, eating the traditional Mediterranean way is a philosophy in itself: Life is for savoring, and food is a glorious and beautiful expression of life. Meals are gatherings of family and friends— genuine events, not inconvenient chores. Food sustains life, and the quality of the food we eat, not to mention the manner and spirit in which it is prepared, is a reflection of the quality of our lives.

In traditional Mediterranean culture, food was both more and less significant than it is in the United States today. Food was less important because it wasn't the source of anxiety we often make it today. Neither was it a commodity, continually reinvented to be faster, cheaper, or lower in fat. Yet, in the Mediterranean, food was and arguably still is far more important than in the United States. Handled and consumed with reverence for its life-sustaining capabilities, food was beautiful, simple, and healthful, a celebration of vitality, loved ones, and life itself.

✎ THE MAGIC DISCOVERED

In the early 1950s, the great American researcher Ancel Keys and his wife, Margaret, were drawn to the southern Italian shores, not just to escape the cold and dark skies of Oxford, England, where Keys was spending a year sabbatical as a visiting professor at Magdalen College, but to explore the curious notion that heart disease was apparently almost nonexistent in this area. At a time when Americans, particularly those in their forties and fifties, were subject to an unusually high rate of heart disease in the United States, Keys was intrigued by reports that the then-new American epidemic was almost unheard of in southern Italy. Heart disease only appeared to occur with any significance within a small upper-class subculture.

Also intriguing were reports of the diet of this region, which was described as nutritionally wholesome but containing very little food from animal products. The diet was low in fat and consisted primarily of plant foods such as vegetables, fruits, and whole grains.

Remember, this was 1950—a time when Americans in general believed large steak dinners, baked potatoes slathered in butter, and a hefty glass of whole milk made a nutritious dinner. How could such a meager, plant-based diet result in such heart-healthy citizens? Keys was compelled to investigate.

Ancel Keys was a revolutionary in the area of nutrition and health. Before Keys, awareness of the link between diet and health was tenuous at best. Keys suspected the link to be more than incidental, and we can credit him with the discovery of the relationship of diet to coronary heart disease. From as early as the 1940s, his clinical work at the University of Minnesota as well as epidemiological observations showed how blood cholesterol was an indicator of heart disease, and that diet—particularly the type of fat consumed—affected blood cholesterol levels. His interest in the relationship of prolonged dietary habits to coronary heart disease rates led him to spearhead one of the greatest and most influential epidemiological studies of our time, the Seven Countries Study.

Keys began his research in Naples, Italy, where he and his wife, Margaret, along with local medical colleagues, studied the blood cholesterol levels and heart disease rates of the local working men. Serum measurements from the initial study subjects revealed extraordinarily low blood cholesterol levels. The male subjects in their forties were especially impressive, with blood cholesterol levels averaging 165 compared to about 230 from blood samples of males of the same age living in Minnesota. As Keys must have suspected, heart disease was rare where cholesterol levels were low.

In his subsequent book *How to Eat Well and Stay Well the Mediterranean Way*, Keys described his results: "What these men told us about their eating habits confirmed dietary studies in the area that reported only about 20 per cent of calories from fats compared with around 40 in Minnesota. According to the doctors who helped us, the hospitals caring for the general populace rarely had coronary heart patients; such patients were found to be only in private clinics caring for the rich."

According to Keys, the diet of the Neapolitan working class was of a quite different composition than the diet consumed by the upper classes, among which meat was consumed daily, as opposed to once every week or two. The diet of the working class sounds both simple and irresistible, as Keys describes it:

The ordinary food of the common Neapolitans consisted of homemade minestrone/vegetable soup, pasta in endless variety, always freshly cooked, served with tomato sauce and a sprinkle of cheese, only occasionally enriched with some bits of meat, or served with a little local seafood without any cheese; a hearty dish of beans and short lengths of macaroni (pasta e fagioli); lots of bread never more than a few hours from the oven and never served with any kind of spread; great quantities of

fresh vegetables; a modest portion of meat or fish
perhaps twice a week; (red) wine; always fresh
fruit for dessert.

Keys states in his book that, when asked years later to formulate a diet that might serve as a preventive against coronary heart disease, he could come up with nothing more suited for this purpose than the traditional working-class diet of early 1950s Naples.

✃ FROM ITALY TO SPAIN AND BEYOND

After their foray into Italy, the Keyses moved on to Spain. The Spanish government was conducting a nutrition survey in Madrid and enlisted Keys and a team of doctors to take and analyze blood samples from a sample of the population in a working-class district called Valle-cas. Compared to Naples, Vallecas was a more impoverished region and the typical diet was even lower in fat, meat, and dairy products than the diets of the Neapolitans. Once again, the incidence of coronary heart disease was exceptionally low, except among the upper class, whose diets were higher in fat from animal sources.

Keys's observations continued. In wealthier Bologna in northern Italy, where the diet is said to be the richest in all of Italy—heavier in cream, butter, and eggs than anywhere else in the country—sure enough, coronary heart disease rates were higher than in Naples (but still far below the rates of coronary heart disease in Boston or Minneapolis). The link was emerging with increasing clarity. In Keys's words: "[saturated] diet fat to blood cholesterol to heart attacks."

Keys continued his explorations, moving on to South Africa, Japan, Hawaii, California, and Finland (the hands-down winner for sky-high cholesterol levels—for more on Finland, see Chapter Three).

The purpose of these investigations was to determine whether an even larger-scale study was warranted, and the results suggested such a study could prove illuminating. The resulting Seven Countries Study was, in fact, not only illuminating, but eventually became one of the most famous and significant of epidemiological studies.

❧ THE SEVEN COUNTRIES STUDY

The plan for the Seven Countries Study was to identify coronary heart disease risk factors and disease rates. In 1958, Keys and his cohorts began examining nearly 13,000 men between the ages of forty and fifty-nine over a five-year period in Greece, Italy, Croatia and Serbia (at the time, both part of Yugoslavia), Japan, Finland, the Netherlands, and the United States. Rather than obtaining data through question-and-answer forms, dietitians were actually stationed in the homes of study subjects, measuring everything eaten and collecting samples to send back to Minnesota for chemical analysis. This type of hands-on data collection resulted in a dietary picture of the study subjects that was probably far more accurate than could ever be obtained via a questionnaire. The extensive study included a follow-up period of an additional ten years on more than 10,000 men and examined a range of lifestyle factors in addition to diet and coronary heart disease rates.

The results of the now famous Seven Countries Study provided strong epidemiological evidence that, indeed, the percentage of calories from saturated fat is linked to increased blood cholesterol levels that result in an increased risk of coronary heart disease. Those countries with the highest consumption of saturated fat, such as the

United States and Finland, had the highest rates of heart disease. The American men participating in the study, as well as the Finnish and Dutch men, had heart disease rates that were twice that of Italian men, and four times that of Greek, Japanese, and Yugoslav men (saturated fat intake was, and still is, comparatively low in Greece, Japan, and Yugoslavia). Furthermore, the study determined that the rates of all-causes, age-specific death rates were among the lowest in the Mediterranean regions.

The Seven Countries Study also identified other key factors that appeared correlated with heart disease. These factors were age, blood pressure, and cigarette smoking. These factors, along with blood cholesterol, came to be known as "universal risk factors" for heart disease. Study after study continued to show that as these factors increased, so did the risk of heart disease. Of all of the identified risk factors, however, blood cholesterol appeared to have the strongest correlation to heart disease.

Although a high saturated-fat diet (which leads to high blood cholesterol levels) may not be, and probably isn't, the sole factor in lower rates of coronary heart disease in the Mediterranean compared with the United States, Keys succinctly states, "The Mediterranean diet is certainly compatible with superior health."

❧ THE INVESTIGATION CONTINUES

Over the past few decades, research study after research study has confirmed the results of the Seven Countries Study: that a diet rich in fruits, vegetables, and whole grains, with low saturated fat, and monounsaturated fat as the primary fat, has been shown repeatedly to be beneficial to health, and to decrease the risk of coronary heart disease and other chronic adult diseases such as diabetes and certain types of cancer. Recently, a study conducted in Lyon, France, led by Michael De Lorgeril, M.D., tested whether a Mediterranean type of diet high in omega-3 fatty acids might reduce the risk of a second heart attack in people who had had a previous heart attack.

The study, which came to be known as the Lyon Diet Heart Study, divided about 600 patients who recently had had a heart attack, were under the age of seventy years old, and suffered no other medical or social ailments, into two groups. The first group, called the experimental group, was placed on a Mediterranean type of diet featuring fish, fruit, cereals, and beans, with about 30 percent of calories from fat. The main source of fat was canola oil, a good source of monounsaturated fat similar to olive oil. Only 8 percent of the calories in this diet was from saturated fat. The diet included about 200 milligrams of cholesterol.

The experimental group was given dietary and lifestyle counseling from health care professionals to ensure compliance. The other group, the control group, were supposedly given general low-fat diet instructions by their physicians to follow.

The study was originally scheduled to run for five years, but after a little over two years, the study was stopped. It appeared that the experimental group, the group consuming the Mediterranean-type diet, had far fewer cardiovascular complications than the control group. Therefore, it was deemed unethical to keep the highly beneficial Mediterranean diet a secret from the control group!

One of the most striking things about this study was that, after the researchers continued to track about 425 of the original study participants for another nineteen months, the original Mediterranean-diet group continued to eat a diet inspired by Mediterranean elements. They liked it that much! And their cardiac health status continued to be much more favorable than those who were not following a Mediterranean-type diet. Patient compliance is often a difficult factor to obtain, so the fact that the experimental group kept eating the prescribed diet even after the study's termination speaks volumes about both the health benefits and, presumably, the enjoyable nature and palatability of a traditional Mediterranean diet.

Research refining the health benefits of various aspects of the Mediterranean diet has been plentiful. The nature of different types of fats has been discovered. For instance, trans-fatty acids—which are found in processed foods containing partially hydrogenated vegetable oils, such as margarine—have been shown to increase heart disease risk. Omega-3 fatty acids, available in fish and from certain vegetable sources like flaxseed, have been shown to decrease the blood's tendency to clot, thereby decreasing heart attack risk. Monounsaturated fats, of which olive oil and canola oil are rich sources, have been shown to increase levels of "good" or HDL cholesterol while lowering "bad" or LDL cholesterol. (For more on fat, see Chapter Three.)

Fat isn't the only component of the Mediterranean diet that seems to be so compatible with good health. The discovery of phytochemicals, the wide array of chemical compounds in plant foods, has prompted a new revolution in nutrition science. The benefits of fiber, antioxidants, and other treasures available to the body through the consumption of plant foods are a continual source of interest to nutrition science. It has become difficult to argue that the Mediterranean diet is anything but conducive to better health and longevity.

Of course, no one nutrient or even a single food group holds the secret to perfect health. Instead, a combination of factors, from fresher and more abundant produce to whole grains and a lower intake of fat from animal sources to a change in attitude, lifestyle, and activity level, seem to contribute to greater heart health, lower cancer risk, and longer life.

The particular "magic" of the traditional Mediterranean diet is just such a combination of factors. Not just monounsaturated fats such as olive oil. Not just whole grains instead of refined. Not just a lower intake of animal products and a higher intake of legumes, nuts, and seeds. Not just fish. Not just the small daily dose of wine with dinner. Instead, all these factors together, resulting in a low overall fat intake with a specific saturated-to-monounsaturated fat ratio, a higher fiber intake, and what amounts to a wide array of phytochemical benefits from a healthy daily dose of plant foods, create a nutritional plan worthy of imitation.

✷ MEDITERRANEAN STYLE: A PHILOSOPHY OF FOOD AND LIFE

Any good scientist knows that research subjects don't exist in a vacuum, and every study runs the risk of producing results influenced by unknown factors. Scientists do their best to minimize the effects of other factors on results, but this isn't always completely possible.

One obvious consideration in examining the lower heart attack rates of people from 1950s and 1960s Mediterranean countries is lifestyle. Today, the effect of the mind on the body is widely publicized and studied (with varying degrees of scientific rigor). Even if a good diet is good for health, could the lifestyle, the stress levels, even the mindset of the people in the Mediterranean contribute to their low coronary disease rates? And what about levels of physical activity?

The Mediterranean lifestyle seems to be as heart-healthy as the Mediterranean diet. We will explore the lifestyle and activity level of the people in the Mediterranean during the 1950s, 1960s, and before. During the postwar era, much of the Mediterranean region was impoverished and didn't advance technologically as the United States did. The area remained largely untouched by technology and all its accompanying developments, relying instead on traditional methods for everything, from farming to cooking.

This translated to a lot more daily physical activity, a greater reliance on family and friends, and a closer daily communion with the natural world. People worked vigorously throughout the day, getting plenty of fresh air and cardiovascular, as well as muscle-strengthening, exercise. Even the Mediterranean sun may have certain health benefits. A recent study reported in the *Tufts University Health & Nutrition Newsletter* revealed that women who live in sunny places were 30 to 40 percent less likely to get breast cancer than women who live in northern areas or those who usually stay inside during the day.

The emphasis on family and a strong support system of friends in small communities probably contributed to lower stress levels, as did a slower pace of living, an appreciation of nature, and not insignificantly, a reverence for the food on the table. Food is an essential component of everyday life in the Mediterranean, not something to grab on the go, not something that comes in a freezer box or a microwaveable packet, but something grown by hand then picked and, within hours, eaten. Food is cooked according to long tradition and savored as the life-giving force it is.

Assessing the benefit of attitudes about life, nature, and food on coronary health is difficult from a scientific point of view. These factors are harder to isolate than dietary components. However, common sense can come into play once again when considering the lifestyle of the people in the Mediterranean. To live well, at a slower pace; to love well and rely on family and friends; to appreciate the natural world by living in it, working it, and harvesting its bounty; and to relish the food on the table each day—this kind of life must certainly be conducive to a long, healthy existence.

ॐ LIVING THE GUIDELINES

The traditional Mediterranean diet may sound pretty good right about now, but how does it compare to every other diet you've recently heard touted on a talk show or in the columns of your favorite health magazine or local newspaper? A steaming plate of pasta laden with fresh vegetables and a fragrant hunk of whole-grain bread for supper tonight sounds great, but how does this compare with the guidelines proposed by the American Heart Association and the American Dietetic Association?

In the next chapter, we will examine in more detail the breakdown of components in the traditional Mediterranean diet, as well as the components of the traditionally recommended American Heart Association diet and several other widely available eating systems recommended by different organizations. We won't send you off to the dinner table without a little more knowledge under your belt.

ॐ QUESTIONS AND ANSWERS

ॐ *Can the Mediterranean diet help with weight loss?*

Certainly! The traditional Mediterranean diet is a low-fat diet high in fiber and containing a wide array of vita-

mins, minerals, and phytochemicals, compatible with
good health and the maintenance of normal body weight.
Many weight-loss plans advocate increased consumption
of vegetables, fruit, and whole grains, with a decreased
consumption of saturated fat. Design your meals to feature fresh produce and whole grains. Use high-fat animal
products only occasionally, deriving daily protein from
beans, low-fat dairy products, moderate amounts of nuts,
and small amounts of low-fat meat for flavoring. Stick to
single portions, and add to that a more active lifestyle.
You should be able to lose weight, if you are overweight,
with relative ease, and at a sensible rate (one to two
pounds per week). Also, if you are trying to lose weight,
you may be better off foregoing that Mediterranean glass
of wine with dinner. Alcohol can stimulate the appetite
and add extra calories. Contacting a registered dietitian
will help determine your individual caloric and nutrient
needs.

℘ *How does one switch over to a more Mediterranean-
style diet without changing eating habits too drastically?*

Moving to a more Mediterranean-influenced diet is an
easy and delicious experience. Gradually replace butter
and margarine with olive oil in dishes—to sauté vegetables, added to soup for flavoring, or to keep pasta from
sticking. Olive oil even works for baking. The distinctive
olive oil flavor disappears during the baking process (or,
if you find olive oil undesirable for baking, try the milder
tasting canola oil). Then, stock up on whole grains,
legumes, pasta, canned tomatoes, and in-season produce,
when available.

Have fun with meal planning, and keep a few guidelines
in mind: Feature fresh fruits, seasonal vegetables, and

wholesome whole grains like rice, cornmeal, and bread at every meal, but keep the butter or margarine off the table.

Get in the habit of using meat for flavoring only, and not at every meal. Many delicious Mediterranean dishes don't use meat at all, and are, consequently, economical as well as delicious. Remember that legumes, nuts, and seeds are excellent sources of protein.

Visit farmer's markets, produce stands, or the produce department at your local grocery store to find the best, freshest seasonal fruits and vegetables available. Remember, to eat Mediterranean is largely a matter of eating what's in season. Jettison the dessert course. If you are in the habit of finishing with something sweet, choose the best, ripest, freshest fruit when available, or dried fruit such as sweet, plump dried figs, dates, or a handful of raisins to satisfy your sweet tooth. Even canned fruit, in its own juice, is preferable to high-fat, high-sugar fare. Although certain Mediterranean desserts may be famous worldwide (baklava from Greece or canoli from Italy, for example), such extravagance is traditionally reserved for special occasions.

Last, if you drink alcohol, try drinking wine, but only with meals and in small amounts. (More on this later.)

Remember the Mediterranean rules: Quality, not quantity. Fresh and whole, not processed and preserved. And most important, relish the experience of eating. Savor every bite.

℀ *What studies have been done on the diets of some of the other Mediterranean countries besides Crete, France, and Italy?*

One study published in the British journal *The Lancet* examined the life expectancy in Albania. Albania is considered the most impoverished European country, with one of the highest infant mortality rates in Europe. Yet, Albanian adults have a life expectancy about equal to that of adults in other central and eastern European countries, and male deaths from coronary heart disease are about the level as those in Italy. Mortality rates were lowest in southwest Albania, along its Mediterranean shore, where people consumed the greatest quantities of olive oil, fruits, and vegetables, and the lowest levels of meat and dairy products. The study concluded that diet was the most likely explanation for Albania's surprisingly low mortality rates, even though reliable dietary information on Albania wasn't available.

℘ *What ingredients and dishes compatible with a healthy diet are characteristic of Mediterranean countries whose cuisines are less well known than those of Spain, France, Italy, and Greece?*

The cuisine of Morocco is distinctive and delicious, including such traditional dishes as tagine (stew), couscous (steamed cracked durum wheat semolina), and kesra (an anise-scented bread). Fresh produce favorites include pumpkin, zucchini, eggplant, potatoes, tangerines, strawberries, Medjool dates, green beans, and bananas. Moroccan cuisine also relies heavily on seafood, sometimes marinated with charmoula, a luscious combination of cumin, paprika, fresh herbs, and lemon juice. Spices characteristic of Moroccan dishes include cumin, paprika, turmeric, Spanish saffron, cinnamon, and ginger. Meals are typically very low in fat and high in fiber, consisting primarily of grains, beans, and fresh vegetables and fruits (dried fruits are sometimes used in stews). Meat, seafood, and poultry are special-occasion ingredients. Meals often end with fruit salad, and dessert usually consists of mint tea made with fresh spearmint, Morocco's national drink.

Algerian food is notoriously spicy with lots of sauces and fish dishes. Meals often start with soup or salad, then feature roast meat as a main course and fruit for dessert. Couscous is an Algerian staple and French bread covered in spicy sauce as well as meat on skewers are available in many food stalls. Alcohol is expensive, and although Algeria produces some wines they are generally not served in the country itself due to the Muslim prohibition of alcohol.

Tunisian cuisine has recently become popular. Tunisians are big fans of hot peppers. Common ingredients in the simple, healthful meals include nuts; olives; fish; olive oil; spiced octopus, squid, and shrimp; shredded greens; carrots; pumpkins; and zucchini. Vegetables and seafood are often blended or served separately with hot peppers, spices, lemon juice, and olive oil. Meals almost always begin with a salad of tomato, lettuce, onion, spices, and olives. Coriander, anise, cumin, and cinnamon are popular spices. Couscous is another mainstay. A fried pastry snack called brik is popular but not a daily part of the traditional diet. Other popular Tunisian specialties include chorba, a peppery soup; chakchouka, a ratatouille with chickpeas, tomatoes, peppers, garlic, and onions served with an egg; and tagine, a thick stew.

Libyan cuisine is much like the cuisines of Algeria and Tunisia. Couscous is a mainstay. Spiced rice with meat and vegetables is a common meal. Libya is a Muslim country as well, and alcohol was banned by the government in 1969.

Egyptian cuisine is influenced by the cuisines of Greece, Turkey, Lebanon, Palestine, and Syria. Common dishes include vegetable stews, rice and pasta, salads, and bread. Some traditional dishes include fried eggplant, mixed or grilled salads often including grilled eggplant, beetroot, potato, mushrooms, chickpeas, blackeyed peas, cauliflower, tahini (sesame butter), artichokes, onions, spinach, and tomatoes; soups made with onion, tomato, yellow lentils, and other vegetables, and a variety of dried bean dishes; mixed dishes of ground meat, rice and lentils with tomato sauce, garlic and potatoes; stuffed grape leaves, walnut sauce, and a variety of breads.

The cuisine of Lebanon has had an incredible influence on the world, considering the country's small size. It is also in line with the components of the traditional Mediterranean diet: whole grains, fruits, vegetables, and seafood. Although chicken and lamb are the most common meats, animal products make up a small portion of the diet. Garlic and olive oil are the primary flavorings, and butter and cream are rarely used. Raw, cooked, and pickled vegetables make up a major part of most meals. Lebanon's national dish is kibbeh, a fresh lamb-and-bulgur wheat paste similar to pâté, and sometimes served with yogurt sauce. Bread is a mainstay, present at every meal, often seasoned with olive oil. Several excellent Lebanese wines are available, but alcohol is always served with food. Like the tapas of Spain and the antipasto of Italy, mezze is a Lebanese collection of appetizers often including pickled vegetables, bread, seafood, and salads, both cooked and raw. Baklava, of Greek origin, is a popular Lebanese dessert. Coffee is served throughout the day, often flavored with cardamom and heavily sweetened. Traditional Lebanese dishes include tabbouleh, a salad of bulgur wheat, parsley, and mint; fattoush, a toasted bread salad; hummus tahini, a paste of chickpeas, sesame butter, olive oil, lemon juice, and parsley; and baba ghanouj, a roasted eggplant puree.

Traditional Turkish food includes many yogurt-based dishes, fish in olive oil, a variety of salads and stuffed vegetables including vine leaves, and the syrupy phyllo-pastry desserts also popular in Greece and other Middle Eastern countries. The Turkish diet is still mostly in conformance with the traditional Mediterranean diet. Turkish vineyards produce wine grapes and yellow sultana raisins. Lamb and chicken are the most popular meats. Fresh ingredients are of primary importance, and produce is typically served seasonally. Bread is a primary part of the Turkish diet. Popular local produce items include eggplants, olives, figs, pistachios, peaches, apricots, and several types of nuts, including pistachios and hazelnuts. Shish kebab and flatbread are two classic Turkish dishes. Popular seasonings include mint, parsley, cinnamon, dill, garlic, pepper flakes, and sumac. Turkish meals often include a *zeytinagli*, or olive oil course, in which various foods are prepared with olive oil. Minced meat dishes and seafood specialties are well known, and fruit is the most common dessert. Although Turkish coffee is famous worldwide, tea is a popular drink. Other traditional Turkish dishes include ashure, a cereal pudding with dried and fresh fruit and nuts; a yogurt drink called ayran; borek, a stuffed pastry; dolma, the term for any stuffed vegetable but most often referring to stuffed grape leaves; manti, a small, ravioli-like, meat-stuffed pastry; sis kofte, or shish kebab; and yufka, a flatbread.

ॐ *How much wine is typically included in the traditional Mediterranean diet?*

Keep in mind that a serving of wine is only about 4 ounces. Many wineglasses available today hold twice that much or more! In Greece, the subject of much research and considered by many the standard against which all Mediterranean diets should be measured, men traditionally drank two or three glasses of wine each day. That only comes to 8 to 12 ounces. Women consumed less, and sometimes none at all. Considering the research that suggests alcohol consumption, even in moderation, could increase breast cancer risk, women should proceed with caution when considering whether to include wine as a part of their diets. Also remember that in general, research has revealed that moderate alcohol consumption is often found to reduce the risk of cardiovascular disease, but at the same time, it increases the risk of some cancers, and also increases the risk of accidents, including motor vehicle accidents.

2: *A Recipe for Wellness*

Have you noticed that almost every time you turn on your television, some authority on something is proclaiming that what we eat, or aren't eating, is negatively impacting our health? From local news broadcasts to tabloid news shows, nutrition is big news these days. What to eat, what not to eat, how much of this or that, eat nothing but this, never ever eat that . . . how did eating ever become so complicated?

Ever since scientists discovered that diet can indeed impact health, people have been excited that they can, indeed, exercise a measure of control over how well they feel, not to mention their chances of developing chronic disease. In response to this excitement, a profusion of "diets of the week" has arisen. Fad diets proclaiming to be a panacea for health problems, weight problems, low energy, inability to concentrate, and on and on, have saturated the media for years. Is the Mediterranean diet just one more fad? Or does it make good sense in terms of the nutritional guidelines familiar to Americans for decades?

Exotic as it sounds, the traditional Mediterranean diet is more than practical and easy to follow. It fits right in with our contemporary way of eating, and the nutritional "laws" we have been taught to follow. Sure, a traditional

Mediterranean diet has its unique qualities—olive oil instead of butter, its own characteristic combinations of herbal flavorings, and recipes combining foods in ways many Americans haven't previously considered. Yet, taken at its core principles, the Mediterranean diet sounds pretty familiar to anyone listening to nutritional advice offered by influential health-related organizations such as the United States Department of Agriculture (USDA), the American Heart Association, and the American Cancer Society. These organizations, and others, have proposed nutritional guidelines and/or food pyramids in the hopes of improving the health of the general population. To get a perspective on where the traditional Mediterranean diet fits in relation to the systems proposed by others, let's examine some of the major nutritional guidelines commonly available. The following describes nutritional advice from some of the more influential of these organizations. As you will see, the Mediterranean diet fits nicely into the parameters of most of these recommendations.

❦ THE AMERICAN HEART ASSOCIATION

The American Heart Association has been actively involved in promoting a heart-healthy diet for decades, from the publication of their popular cookbook first issued in the early 1970s to an extensive, user-friendly web site. Back in 1957, the AHA proposed that a reduction in dietary fat intake would result in a reduction of coronary heart disease, which was already the leading cause of disability and death in the United States and in other developed countries as well.

The AHA continues to issue policy statements relating to the link between diet and coronary heart disease, modifying and updating their position as necessary in response to the latest research. The AHA's position remains consistent, however, when it comes to fat consumption: too much fat, especially saturated fat, increases the risk of coronary heart disease.

In an attempt to help Americans prevent heart and blood vessel disease, the American Heart Association has issued dietary guidelines to promote heart-healthy nutrition. In 1989, nine health and government organizations, including the AHA, met to review the latest scientific findings, and concluded that a few specific dietary changes could maintain and/or improve the health of most Americans. In 1996, the AHA guidelines officially included lifestyle goals, such as quitting cigarette smoking.

The American Heart Association Eating Plan for Healthy Americans is as follows. Note the percentages provided below are to be averaged over a week, rather than applied to single foods or even a day's worth of food, to encourage a variety of foods in the diet:

- Saturated fatty acid intake should be 8 to 10 percent of total calories.
- Polyunsaturated fatty acid intake should be up to 10 percent of total calories.
- Monounsaturated fatty acids should make up to 15 percent of total calories.
- Cholesterol intake should be less than 300 milligrams per day.
- Sodium intake should be less than 2,400 milligrams per day, which is about 1¼ teaspoons of salt.
- Carbohydrate intake should make up 55 to 60 percent or more of calories, with emphasis on increasing sources of complex carbohydrates (like whole grains) as opposed to refined carbo-

hydrates (such as foods that contain a lot of refined sugars).

• Total calories should be adjusted to achieve and maintain a healthy body weight.

Although the AHA guidelines don't mention specific foods, the nutrient proportions are compatible with the traditional Mediterranean diet, as one might expect, considering the research linking a traditional Mediterranean diet with such dramatically low coronary heart disease rates.

℅ THE AMERICAN CANCER SOCIETY

According to the American Cancer Society (ACS), about 500,000 people die from cancer in the United States each year, and about one third of these deaths are due to dietary factors. (Another third can be attributed to cigarette smoking.) It is only natural, then, that the American Cancer Society would publish its own set of nutritional guidelines. If behavioral factors like diet have a significant influence on cancer risk, that's good news! Behavioral factors, unlike genetic factors, are largely within our control. A healthy diet, coupled with physical activity and other lifestyle changes, can go a long way toward reducing cancer risk.

Not surprisingly, the ACS's dietary guidelines are also in line with the traditional Mediterranean diet. They include a high proportion of plant foods in the diet, limited consumption of high-fat foods, and a sensible balance of caloric intake and physical activity. The specific ACS dietary guidelines, as formulated by the ACS Advisory Committee on Diet, Nutrition, and Cancer Prevention in 1996 (and reaffirmed by the ACS Advisory Group on Diet, Physical Activity, and Cancer in 1998), are as follows:

- Choose most of the foods you eat from plant sources.
- Limit your intake of high-fat foods, particularly from animal sources.
- Be physically active and achieve and maintain a healthy weight.
- Limit consumption of alcoholic beverages, if you drink at all.

❧ THE UNITED STATES DEPARTMENT OF AGRICULTURE

The United States Department of Agriculture (USDA) formulated the Dietary Guidelines for Americans in 1995. Many organizations, such as the American Dietetic Association, endorse these guidelines as a healthful way to eat and a proactive approach to chronic disease prevention.

The Dietary Guidelines for Americans are provided below. They, too, are quite compatible with the traditional Mediterranean diet:

- Eat a variety of foods. (The traditional Mediterranean diet celebrates culinary diversity, eating according to what is freshest and seasonally available, resulting in a wide sampling of foods from both land and sea.)
- Choose a diet with plenty of grain products, vegetables, and fruits. (These food groups form the basis of the traditional Mediterranean diet.)
- Choose a diet low in fat, saturated fat, and cholesterol. (Because so few animal products are

consumed in the traditional Mediterranean diet, it is low in saturated fat and cholesterol. Even though olive oil consumption is high in some areas, total fat intake is still typically below that of the average American.)

- Choose a diet moderate in salt and sodium. (Very few traditional Mediterranean recipes add salt.)
- Choose a diet moderate in sugars. (Sugary desserts are special treats, not a daily part of the traditional Mediterranean diet.)
- Balance the food you eat with physical activity—maintain or improve your weight. (The people living the traditional Mediterranean lifestyle are typically very active in their daily lives, working as farmers or engaging in other physical labor.)
- If you drink alcoholic beverages, do so in moderation. (Although the traditional Mediterranean diet often includes wine with every meal except breakfast, portions are small and alcohol is typically consumed only with food, not recreationally.)

The USDA also formulated the Food Guide Pyramid, which has been widely distributed and can be found on the packaging of many ready-to-eat foods, such as on cereal boxes. The pyramid was created in 1992, as updated nutritional advice meant to replace the four food groups the government had previously espoused. In conjunction with the Department of Health and Human Services, the USDA developed its Food Guide Pyramid to be a visual representation of how much of what types of foods should be eaten, on average, each day. The pyramid shape was chosen because it clearly depicts the foods that should be eaten in greatest quantity each day at the widest part of the pyramid, working up to foods that should be eaten only sparingly at the apex.

Food Guide Pyramid

A Guide to Daily Food Choices

Fats, Oils, & Sweets
USE SPARINGLY

KEY
□ Fat (naturally occurring and added)   ▨ Sugars (added)
These symbols show that fat and added sugars come mostly from fats, oils, and sweets, but can be part of or added to foods from the other food groups as well.

Milk, Yogurt, & Cheese Group
2-3 SERVINGS

Meat, Poultry, Fish, Dry Beans, Eggs, & Nuts Group
2-3 SERVINGS

Vegetable Group
3-5 SERVINGS

Fruit Group
2-4 SERVINGS

Bread, Cereal, Rice, & Pasta Group
6-11 SERVINGS

SOURCE: U.S. Department of Agriculture / U.S. Department of Health and Human Services.

The pyramid has met with praise as well as criticism. One of the biggest critics of the USDA's Food Guide Pyramid is the Oldways Preservation and Exchange Trust.

❀ EATING THE "OLDWAYS" WAY

The Oldways Preservation and Exchange Trust may not be familiar to the public, but this nonprofit, Cambridge, Massachusetts-based organization has been highly influential in the dissemination of information about the benefits of the traditional Mediterranean diet. This group seeks to resurrect many of the "old ways" of eating before the advent of food processing, and they have published guidelines for eating in the traditional Mediterranean way. Among these guidelines is their own version of the Food Guide Pyramid, the Mediterranean Food Guide Pyramid.

The Traditional Healthy Mediterranean Diet Pyramid

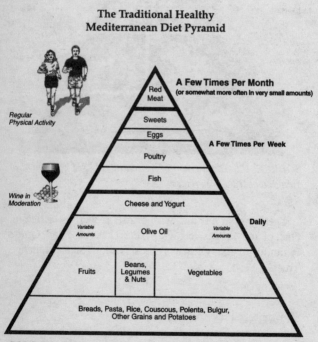

Red Meat — **A Few Times Per Month** (or somewhat more often in very small amounts)

Regular Physical Activity

Sweets

Eggs — **A Few Times Per Week**

Poultry

Fish

Wine in Moderation

Cheese and Yogurt

Daily

Variable Amounts — Olive Oil — *Variable Amounts*

Fruits | Beans, Legumes & Nuts | Vegetables

Breads, Pasta, Rice, Couscous, Polenta, Bulgur, Other Grains and Potatoes

SOURCE: Oldways Preservation and Exchange Trust, Cambridge, MA; 1994.

Citing a recognition of high adult life expectancy rates and low chronic disease rates in the Mediterranean region around 1960, knowledge of food typically consumed in the area during this time, and the compatibility of these eating patterns with current knowledge of nutrition science, Oldways has developed a list of Characteristics of Traditional Healthy Mediterranean Diets that make the diet sound anything but exotic:

- A diet centered on foods from plant sources: vegetables, fruits, whole grains, bread, pasta, nuts, and seeds
- Focus on foods that are locally grown and minimally processed
- Olive oil as the primary source of fat
- Total fat consumption between 25 percent to over 35 percent of calories with no more than 7 to 8 percent of calories from saturated fat
- Daily consumption of low to moderate amounts of cheese and/or yogurt (preferably low fat or nonfat)
- Weekly consumption of low to moderate amounts of fish and poultry (with an emphasis on fish)
- No more than four eggs per week, including those used in cooking and baking
- Fresh fruit as a typical dessert; high-sugar and/or high-fat desserts no more than a few times per week
- Red meat only a few times per month (no more than 12 to 16 ounces or 340 to 450 grams per month)
- Regular physical activity to promote a healthy weight and overall fitness
- Moderate wine consumption with meals (although Oldways now emphasizes this is an optional component, not appropriate for everyone)

These guidelines give a simple overview of trends in the general Mediterranean diet. According to Oldways, the widely circulated United States Department of Agriculture (USDA) dietary guidelines and their Food Guide Pyramid have not made enough of an impact on the public health profile in the United States.

✿ THE PYRAMID SCHEME

The USDA Food Guide Pyramid is the most widely circulated of the pyramids, but other organizations, such as the Oldways Preservation and Exchange Trust and the American Heart Association (AHA), publish their own versions of food pyramids. (We have not included the AHA pyramid in this book because it is not as widely distributed as the USDA pyramid.) These pyramids are similar, but certain important differences exist as well. And, because all these pyramids have their important aspects but also include elements we believe could be improved, we will add our own pyramid to the mix, the Mediterranean Diet Pyramid.

While we feel the advice contained within the other guidelines and pyramids is good, sensible, and conducive to health, we find that the pyramids themselves—the visual representations of the guidelines—tend to be less than user-friendly, sometimes vague, sometimes complicated, and not necessarily updated to reflect the latest research.

Enter the Mediterranean Diet Pyramid. We have developed this pyramid to include what we feel is missing from the others and to include helpful information based on the most cutting-edge research findings on the Mediterranean diet. This pyramid is simply a guideline, not meant to be taken as dietary dogma. It represents a modernized approach to the traditional Mediterranean diet that we believe is user-friendly and compatible with

Our Mediterranean Diet Food Guide Pyramid

Olive oil (or canola oil, but preferably olive oil) drizzled on top

High saturated fat meats, pastries, candy, etc. coconut, margarine, butter,

Other vegetable seed oils, 1 TBS per serving

Monthly (if at all)

Other lean red meats, 1-3 oz. cooked serving

"Lower-fat" cheeses, such as mozzarella made with skim milk

Lean Pork 1-3 oz. cooked serving

Eggs, 4 or less

Veal, 1-3 oz. cooked serving

Low-fat sweets

Weekly (optional, except fish)

Skinless poultry, 1-3 oz. cooked serving

Fish, 6-8 oz. cooked, total for the week

Regular Physical Activity

Nuts and seeds, 1 oz. or more (approximately 1/3 c. nuts)

Low-fat or nonfat dairy, 2 or more servings (8 oz. skim milk, 6 oz. low-fat yogurt, or 1 oz. low-fat cheese)

Daily

Rest & Relaxation

Legumes (Beans, peas), 2 or more 1/2 c. servings

Time with family & friends

Fruit, 2 or more servings (Whole fruit, preferably, instead of processed juice)

Vegetables, 3 or more servings (1/2 c. cooked or 1 c. raw leafy green vegetables)

Whole grains, 8 or more servings

*H/S = Herbs and spices

The Mediterranean Diet Pyramid is intended to show general guidelines. Those with special nutrient needs, such as children, pregnant or lactating women, or those with special dietary requirements, should seek the guidance of a registered dietician or other qualified health care provider for their individual nutrient requirements.

the tastes, habits, and food availability in the United States today. We hope you will find it a useful guide as you begin to alter your dietary patterns to reflect the Mediterranean way.

At first glance, the three pyramids may look similar. However, as mentioned before, we felt the other pyramids to be less than user-friendly as guides to the traditional Mediterranean diet. Our pyramid is a general guideline to help modern Americans eat in a more healthy, traditional Mediterranean way. How is our pyramid different than the other two? The highlights of our pyramid are as follows:

- The Mediterranean Diet Pyramid categorizes foods with clearer distinction. The USDA pyramid has been criticized for lumping foods together that really should be distinguished. For example, meat, poultry, fish, dry beans, eggs, and nuts are listed together. Many of these options are low-fat, healthy choices, but others are high-fat (or more importantly, high in saturated fat), less desirable options that should be consumed far less often than two to three times per day. Although the Oldways pyramid provides more food categories, we hope that we have provided even clearer distinctions.

- The Mediterranean Diet Pyramid lists not only the recommended number of servings to be eaten daily within each category, but how you should structure your diet over the course of a day, a week, and a month. For example, within the daily section, whole grains in the form of breads, pasta, cereals, and so on should be eaten the most (hence their placement at the bottom of the pyramid) in eight or more servings daily. How much you eat in total depends on your individual caloric needs. Consultation with a registered dietitian or other qualified health care provider would be helpful in determining your unique caloric and nutrient needs.

- The "Daily" food section of the Mediterranean Diet Pyramid highlights those plant foods that have been found to be beneficial to health, and in what proportions they can be consumed. As mentioned above, whole grains in the form of breads, cereals, pasta, and so on should be eaten the most in a traditional Mediterranean diet (as also recommended by Oldways and the USDA). You should aim for at least eight servings or more per day. Next, vegetables should be consumed in at least three daily servings. Two or more servings of fruit should also be included daily. An additional cup or more of legumes, as well as 1 ounce or more of nuts and/or seeds should be enjoyed daily. All of these foods contain ample amounts of health-promoting fiber, phytochemicals, vitamins, and minerals. The only food group in the "daily" section that is not from a plant source is the low- or nonfat dairy product group. Some dairy, principally in the form of cheese and yogurt, is a part of the traditional Mediterranean diet, albeit mostly in small amounts. To make our dairy recommendation compatible with heart health, we suggest low- or nonfat dairy foods be included daily for adequate calcium and protein intakes without undesirable excess saturated fat. Notice that lower-fat cheeses, such as mozzarella made from part-skim milk, were placed in the weekly section to be consumed in moderate amounts (1 to 3 ounces total for the week—see Chapter Seven for more on dairy foods), which is still compatible with heart health and in keeping with the traditional Mediterranean spirit.
- The Mediterranean Diet Pyramid separates protein foods in more distinct categories. As men-

tioned, legumes primarily, followed by low- or nonfat dairy foods, and then nuts and seeds should be your daily protein providers. Animal meats should be considered as weekly meal enhancers, rather than the main daily protein source.

- The Mediterranean Diet Pyramid further categorizes different animal meats according to their saturated fat content. Fish, which contains the lowest amount of saturated fat among animal meats, should be eaten the most frequently, up to 6 to 8 cooked ounces total for the week. This more frequent inclusion is also because some fish, particularly the fattier fish like salmon, mackerel, and herring, contain omega-3 fatty acids (more on the health benefits of the omega-3s later). Next on the upward climb on the pyramid is skinless poultry, followed by veal, lean pork, and then lean red meat (such as extra-lean ground beef, tenderloin, and sirloin). High-fat red meat (such as regular ground beef or prime rib) sits at the top of the pyramid and should only be consumed once a month, if at all. Eggs sit on the periphery of the weekly animal list. Moderate intakes of eggs (four or fewer per week) is in keeping with the heart-healthy Mediterranean-inspired eating plan.

Of course, consuming all of the "weekly" animal food sources within a week's time is not likely, and not in keeping with the traditional Mediterranean diet (unless you eat just 1 ounce of each meat category each day, which can get tedious). In addition to the weekly recommendation of fish (we recommend that you strive to include fish in your weekly consumption), one or two of the other animal meats can be included in a week's meal plan, if at all. Certainly, a week without animal meat is also fine and in the spirit of the traditional Mediterranean diet. Just be sure to include plenty of other plant protein sources, and you're in for a heart-healthy week.

- The Mediterranean Diet Pyramid also separates fats and oils in more distinct categories. Olive oil, the Mediterranean culinary star, should be the principal source of fat, followed by canola oil. These oils are high in monounsaturated fats and appear to promote heart health. Butter (high in saturated fat), margarine (which can be high in trans fatty acids), and other vegetable oils should be used on a monthly basis in a truly Mediterranean-inspired diet. Note that olive and canola oil are "drizzled" over the top, not poured. This is because all oils and fats are high in calories, and how much you drizzle depends on your individual caloric needs.

- The Mediterranean Diet Pyramid places highly refined and processed desserts and pastries, which contain large amounts of saturated fat and calories, at the top to show that there is little room for these foods in a traditional Mediterranean eating plan. Candy is another food that lacks nutrients and should be reserved for monthly treats. (Dried fruit makes for a delicious and in many ways a more satisfying daily sweet treat. In fact, fruit should serve as the basis of the majority of desserts and sweets consumed.) To be realistic and in keeping with the American love for sweets, however, we placed low-fat sweets (such as some ready-to-eat cereal bars that do not contain partially hydrogenated oils), and pure, not artificial, sweeteners (such as brown sugar, molasses, pure maple syrup) to be consumed moderately on a weekly basis, if at all.

- Herbs and spices, designated in the pyramid as H/S, are "sprinkled" throughout the Mediterranean Diet Pyramid to emphasize their importance in our recommended eating plan. After all, herbs and spices are plant-derived foodstuffs, and they also contain beneficial phytochemicals. (Even though only small amounts of herbs and spices are usually used at one time, if you use them often enough, the benefits are there.) Indeed, a plant-based Mediterranean-style diet would not be the same without utilizing these items. Who needs a lot of excess salt when herbs and spices such as oregano, parsley, thyme, rosemary, black pepper (the list is endless) are used? Likewise, who needs a lot of excess sugar when cinnamon, cardamom, nutmeg, vanilla and other flavors can bring satisfaction and a feeling of wholesomeness for any sweet lover?

- Outside of the Mediterranean Diet Pyramid are important lifestyle indicators to remind our readers of the important role of regular physical activity (Oldways also indicates this in their pyramid), rest and relaxation, as well as social interaction (especially at mealtime) for overall health. All of these lifestyle attributes, in addition to diet, most likely contributed to the healthier hearts seen in those living in the traditional Mediterranean regions.

- Unlike the Oldways Mediterranean pyramid, we did not highlight wine in our pyramid. We've chosen not to include wine, as we feel it is an optional component. We feel that the foods

emphasized in our pyramid are so beneficial to
health that if wine were omitted, it would not be
missed.

In the following chapters, we will discuss all of the different Mediterranean Diet Pyramid food categories in
more detail.

In the Mediterranean Diet Pyramid, the best elements
of both the USDA and Oldways pyramids have been
combined, along with other elements to make it even
more user-friendly, such as serving sizes and more food
groups, to fully distinguish between foods within certain
groups in terms of nutritional value and recommended
frequency of consumption.

That does not mean, of course, that you must, or even
should, follow it precisely, or all the time. This pyramid
is only a general guideline meant to promote a varied,
low-fat diet compatible with good health. We hope it
will remind you that many, many healthy foods exist out
there from which you can choose and still be within the
Mediterranean spirit of eating. With all the conflicting
nutritional information available, it is easy to become
confused. In the simple and down-to-earth spirit of traditional Mediterranean culture, however, we suggest
that common sense may be the best indicator of action.
Choose a diet that tastes great, is low in fat, high in
fiber, includes sufficient micronutrients, and makes you
feel fantastic. We've found that the traditional Mediterranean diet, with sensible modifications, fits the bill perfectly. And what better reminder of just how healthy,
diverse, delicious, and easy this diet can be than the
visual representation provided by the Mediterranean
Diet Pyramid?

❦ QUESTIONS AND ANSWERS

❦ In general, what counts as a serving?

The Mediterranean Diet Pyramid lists serving sizes in each of its food categories. The USDA also publishes a list of serving sizes for a variety of food groups. In general, however, one serving from the grain group equals one slice of bread. Note that by "slice of bread," we are referring to the standard 70-calorie portion size. If the whole-grain bread you are consuming is labeled with more calories than this per slice, please adjust accordingly. For example, some prepackaged whole-grain breads contain 130 calories per slice, which would really be each equal to two Mediterranean Diet grain servings. A serving is also equal to 1 ounce of ready-to-eat cereal or ½ cup of cooked grains, including rice, pasta, or cooked cereal. This serving is fairly small. Drop a half-cup of pasta on a plate and you'll see what we mean. The small serving size (by American standards, where we have become accustomed to "super-sizing" our meals) puts the USDA's six to eleven serving recommendation from the grain group in perspective. Even eight servings sounds like a lot, but eat a moderate-size bowl of cereal for breakfast, one sandwich for lunch, and one cup of pasta for dinner and you're there.

For the vegetable group, 1 cup of raw leafy vegetables or ½ cup of chopped or cooked other vegetables or ¾ cup of vegetable juice equals a serving. One medium piece of fruit or ½ cup of chopped or cooked fruit, or ½ to ¾ cup of most fruit juices equals a fruit serving. In the dairy category, 1 cup of milk or yogurt or 1.5 ounces of cheese equals a serving, and in the protein group, 2 to 3 ounces of cooked lean meat equals a serving. Note:

One egg, 2 tablespoons of peanut butter, ⅓ cup of most nuts, or ½ cup of cooked lentils equals an ounce of meat.

✿ Does the Mediterranean diet provide enough daily protein for the average adult?

Yes! The Recommended Daily Allowance (RDA) for the average adult male (age twenty-five and up) is 63 grams. For the average adult female (age twenty-five and up and who is not pregnant or lactating), the RDA for protein is 50 grams. If you eat the minimum daily Mediterranean Diet recommendation of 1 cup of legumes (such as chickpeas and red kidney beans) per day, you'll be eating roughly 14 grams of protein. Add in ⅓ cup of nuts (such as walnuts) and you'll be consuming 7 grams more. Consume at least three servings of vegetables (such as green beans and carrots), and you are adding about 3 more grams of protein. Two cups of nonfat dairy equals roughly 16 grams of protein. Eat at least eight servings of whole grains (such as whole-grain bread, couscous, etc.), and you are adding about 24 grams of protein. This already puts us up to 63 grams of protein, and we haven't even left the minimum recommendations of the "daily" food section of the Mediterranean Diet Pyramid. Toss in an ounce of fish (such as tuna) and you'll be getting about 7 more grams of protein.

✿ Can a vegetarian eat a Mediterranean diet?

The traditional Mediterranean diet is almost a lacto-ovo vegetarian diet. While both Mediterranean diet pyramids list meat, poultry, and fish to be consumed any-where from weekly to a few times per month, these items are not, by any means, required. The traditional Mediter-ranean diet is centered around plant foods, with small amounts of cheese and yogurt (depending on the country of a recipe's origin). Many people living in the Mediter-ranean during the 1950s and 1960s probably were vege-tarian, either by choice or by necessity.

Even a vegan (someone who consumes no animal products at all) can follow the traditional Mediterranean diet. Cheese, yogurt, and milk, though all healthy addi-tions to a heart-healthy eating plan, aren't required. Veg-ans must be even more careful to eat food from a wide variety of sources, however, to ensure that all the nutri-tional bases are covered. Vegans might also consider tak-ing supplements, particularly of vitamin B_{12}, which is most available from animal sources. Of course, anyone who eliminates an entire food group from his or her diet should seek the counsel of a registered dietitian to ensure that the proportions of food they do eat are sufficient to meet all nutrient and caloric needs.

�; Is the Mediterranean Diet Pyramid appropriate for children? What about pregnant or breastfeeding women? What about teenagers?

Yes! The Mediterranean diet, when eaten in correct proportions and sufficient amounts, is nutritionally ade-quate for anyone. Again, however, we recommend that you contact a registered dietitian if you have any special nutritional and/or caloric needs such as those of a grow-ing child or a pregnant or breastfeeding woman.

❧ *Can someone with a chronic disease such as diabetes or kidney disease safely eat a Mediterranean diet?*

People with chronic diseases have unique nutritional and/or caloric needs, so again, we recommend contacting a registered dietitian about the diet that is right for the individual. Certain food items or groups may be prohibited for you. Although you may have to customize certain elements according to your needs, in general, a Mediterranean diet is a healthy, nutrient-dense diet appropriate for anyone able to eat it.

❧ *Are vitamin, mineral, or other dietary supplements necessary or beneficial while following the traditional Mediterranean diet?*

No, the nutrient-dense Mediterranean diet provides all essential nutrients when eaten in sufficient quantities (as depicted in the Mediterranean Diet Pyramid). If you suspect you aren't deriving adequate nutrition from your diet or if you have special nutritional needs, seek the advice of a registered dietitian.

❧ *Why does the American Heart Association recommend averaging percentages, such as the 30-percent-of-calories-from-fat rule, over a few days or a week rather than on a daily basis?*

In the words of the AHA, "Applying the 30 percent standard to single foods greatly limits the variety of foods in the diet and can be misleading. The only way to maintain balance, variety and enjoyment of the AHA eating plan is to interpret the guideline with emphasis on the words 'total calories.' " In other words, occasionally it makes sense to have a day where calories from fat will exceed 30 percent. If days like this are balanced with days where total calories from fat fall below 30 percent, this is more conducive to a varied (and interesting) diet. For more on the AHA recommendations, check out the "Dietary Guidelines for Healthy American Adults," available on the AHA web site: http://americanheart.org/Heart_and_Stroke_A_A_Guide/dlietg.html.

❧ Which dairy products besides nonfat or low-fat milk are a sensible addition to a low-fat diet?

A wide variety of low-fat and nonfat yogurts are available. The kind without added sugar is preferable. Stir in some fresh fruit for sweetness. Also, while some cheeses are very high in fat, others are relatively low in fat. Check the labels, or look for cheeses made from skim milk (such as mozzarella made with part-skim milk). Pretty much all of the cheeses come in reduced or nonfat versions. Cottage cheese, ricotta, feta, gouda, Cheddar—the list seems endless—are now offered in reduced-fat or nonfat varieties.

❧ Where does high-fat cheese fit into the Mediterranean Diet Pyramid?

High-fat cheeses (such as Gruyère, muenster, blue) are full of flavor, so a little goes a long way. Although a dairy product, high-fat cheese is more appropriately located with high-fat meats as a high-fat protein source. If you like them, consume high-fat cheese only every month or so and in small amounts.

❦ Canned beans are much easier to prepare than dried beans. Are they just as healthy?

Yes. For those that are salt-sensitive, however, be careful about the excess sodium. Rinse canned beans in a colander to wash away the salt. Rinsing will also wash away some of the starchy liquid, making your dishes more attractive, as well as reducing the likelihood of developing intestinal gas after bean consumption. If the recipe in which you are using canned beans calls for added salt (not often the case with traditional Mediterranean recipes), you might consider adjusting the added salt accordingly.

❦ Are certain nuts and seeds better than others?

From a nutritional point of view, all nuts and seeds are nutrient-dense plant foods. Some are lower in fat than others, however, and consequently lower in calories, so these nuts and seeds might be more appropriate for people who are attempting to control their weight. Chestnuts are actually a low-fat food. A 1-ounce serving of roasted (European) chestnuts (about three and a half nuts) contains less than 1 gram of fat, all unsaturated, and about 70 calories. On the opposite end of the scale, 1 ounce of dry-roasted cashews contains about 13 grams of fat and 163 calories, and 1 ounce of toasted or roasted sesame seeds contains about 14 grams of fat and 160 calories. The key is to get a variety of nuts and seeds to benefit most from the varied nutrients and phytochemicals (more on this later). The more variety, the healthier the diet really is. Of course, eating that variety in moderation is important, too.

Coconuts are a rare exception to the heart-healthy plant food rule. Coconuts are high in saturated fat and are best avoided most of the time.

❦ *The Mediterranean Diet Pyramid lists "four or fewer" eggs at the "weekly" level. Is it okay to eat more eggs if only the whites are consumed?*

Yes, by all means. Egg whites do not contain cholesterol, which is found only in the yolks. They are a good source of protein and can be used to cut fat in egg dishes and baked dishes as well. Also, research supports the notion that consumption of saturated fat, not dietary cholesterol (sometimes called preformed cholesterol), has the most impact on blood cholesterol levels. While some people are very sensitive to dietary cholesterol and should limit egg consumption, the general population need not be overly concerned about dietary cholesterol. The "four or fewer per week" egg rule is just a general guideline for a Mediterranean-inspired (or any nutritionally sound) eating program.

❦ *How can someone lose weight putting olive oil on everything?*

We certainly don't recommend putting olive oil on everything! Olive oil is fat, and fat in excess contributes to obesity, which in turn contributes to many health problems. One common misconception about the Mediterranean diet is that adding olive oil to an already high-fat diet will "fix" the fat problem. On the contrary, olive oil should substitute for other types of fat, not be added to them. Overall fat intake from all sources, including olive oil, should be lower than is typical for Americans. This is why we recommend "drizzling" olive oil, not pouring it, over our visual representation of a healthy Mediterranean-inspired diet. A little goes a long way.

✤ Are some vegetables better choices than others? What about fruits?

All fruits and vegetables (in fact, all plant foods, with the exception of coconut and palm oils—more on these in Chapter Three) have their "star" qualities. Also, every type of plant food has a unique combination of nutrients and phytochemicals. That's why a variety of plant foods is more important than choosing a few "right" plant foods and eating only those. The more variety in your diet, the more nutritionally complete your diet will be.

✤ What about table sugar? Is sugar an acceptable addition to a healthy, Mediterranean diet?

The sugar controversy rages on. Some people proclaim it as among the worst possible additions to your diet. Others say that, as long as a person maintains a healthy weight and sufficient nutrients are consumed, sugar is fine. The truth probably lies somewhere in the middle. Whenever you eat a high-sugar product, you are filling up with empty calories when you could have eaten something more nutrient-dense instead. If you are getting enough to eat but add sugar, you may have trouble maintaining that ideal weight. But, if consumed occasionally in moderation, as part of a healthy diet, sugar is probably just fine—and pretty hard to avoid these days.

✤ What about coffee and tea?

Although not listed on either Mediterranean food pyramid, coffee and/or tea are both integral—albeit nonnutritive—parts of the diets in many Mediterranean countries. In fact, it would be difficult to discuss the Mediterranean region without mentioning the infamous Italian espresso, not to mention the thick, sweet, sludgy concoction known as Turkish coffee. Tea is also widely consumed in many Mediterranean countries. However, we suggest that if you enjoy coffee and/or tea, you consume them in moderation like anything else, and not at the expense of more nutritionally complete foods. Also, if you are caffeine-sensitive, we recommend discussing the use of caffeine with your physician.

✤ Is canola oil just as good as olive oil?

Canola oil is, by necessity, more processed than olive oil. Therefore, it loses many of the vital phytochemical components still present in extra-virgin olive oil. However, it is a good source of monounsaturated fat and it is generally cheaper than olive oil. For more information on fat in general and olive and canola oil in particular, see Chapter Three.

✤ Can the Mediterranean Diet Pyramid be used as a guide for non-Mediterranean types of cuisine?

Yes! The idea is to apply the Mediterranean concept, not necessarily the particular food ingredients, to all your food choices. You need not limit yourself to pasta primavera, for example. Instead, base your diet around plant foods, focusing on vegetables, whole grains, fruit, primarily beans for protein, and animal meat in moderation. This goal works for just about any cuisine. In fact, bar-and-grill-type American restaurants often have grilled vegetable entrées. Most restaurants have salads with small amounts of meat such as grilled chicken on top. Ask for olive oil and vinegar as a dressing and you've got a great Mediterranean-inspired meal!

Asian cuisine is right in line with the principles of traditional Mediterranean cuisine. Who can deny the proclaimed health benefits of soy foods such as tofu? Rice and vegetables with protein from small amounts of meat or tofu (a cheeselike soybean curd) or nuts and seeds (peanut sauce, walnuts, almonds, cashews, and peanuts are common Asian additions) make an exceptionally healthy meal.

Even an American home barbecue can fit in with the Mediterranean concept if you fill up on green salad, baked beans, coleslaw made with vinaigrette instead of mayonnaise, grilled or raw vegetables, and fruit such as watermelon and fresh fruit salad. You probably won't even miss the burger and hot dogs!

❧ The Mediterranean Diet Pyramid seems to require a lot of food be consumed, especially in the daily food section. Will I gain weight?

No, not very likely, especially if you incorporate daily activity into your schedule. If you consume the minimum requirement of each of the recommended daily food groups, you will be consuming about 1,385 calories. Add in a tablespoon of olive oil, and you are still only talking about (roughly) 1,500 calories. Factor in a 3-ounce cooked portion of fish, such as salmon, and you're adding around 200 calories, for a total of 1,700 calories for the day. The average adult can easily maintain weight on such a diet. In fact, many people will lose weight on any diet below 1,800 calories, especially those who are moderately active.

The Mediterranean diet really should not be about numbers. Rather, the culinary spirit of the traditional Mediterranean region should be celebrated and enjoyed for the many benefits it possesses. Again, if your health requires you to gain or lose weight, you should seek the guidance of a registered dietitian or other qualified health care provider for your individual needs. Our pyramid should act only as a general guide to shape your eating habits to closely resemble the healthy traditional Mediterranean diet.

3: Olive Oil and Other Fats: What You Need to Know

⊕ *Fat.* Does the word make you cringe? Fat is bad, bad, bad . . . isn't it? Eating fat makes us overweight, gives us heart attacks, causes cancer, wrecks our health . . . doesn't it? If it says "fat free," it must be healthy . . . isn't that true?

Yet, if fat is so bad, how is it that in certain Mediterranean regions such as the Greek island of Crete during the 1950s, where heart disease and other chronic disease rates were startlingly low, fat consumption was about equal to fat consumption in America? Cretans during this time in history were among the longest-lived people in the world. Yet, their diet was full of fat.

According to researcher Ancel Keys, Cretans consumed 3 to 4 ounces (or about ½ cup) of olive oil *per day, per person.* That's a lot of fat! Keys reported that the people of Crete drenched their salads in it, dunked their bread in it, poured it on their potatoes. Some Cretan farmers even drank a wineglass full of the stuff for breakfast! Why weren't the people on this tiny island suffering from the same health problems as Americans during the 1950s and '60s, those health problems we've been told had (and still have) everything to do with too much fat in our diets?

Perhaps Crete is an anomaly? Yet, studies from other countries reveal similarly striking results. Heart disease rates in the southern, or rather the Mediterranean, regions of Italy, Spain, and France were also remarkably low, even though percentage of fat calories varied greatly around the region.

Yet, not every country could get away with fat consumption to the degree enjoyed in the Mediterranean. Keys's studies of fat consumption and diet also included Finland, the country with the most coronary heart disease and the shortest life spans in Europe. Keys examined middle-aged men in Finland to determine why coronary heart disease was so common in this country, even among men who were thinner and more physically fit than many of the overweight, less fit American men in Keys's studies. Blood cholesterol levels of the Finnish men proved to exceed average levels in American men.

Subsequent dietary surveys revealed that the typical diet in Finland was extremely high in saturated fat. According to Keys, meals included "great mounds of butter" and it was not unusual to see "grown men down a couple of glasses of rich milk." Keys also relates watching Finnish loggers take "slabs of cheese the size of slices of sandwich bread, smear them a quarter of an inch deep with butter and eat them with a beer as an after-sauna snack."

Other studies conducted by Keys revealed that among patients with very high blood cholesterol levels, diets very low in fat produced dramatic drops in cholesterol levels within one week, and studies examining the effects of different types of fatty acids—saturated, monounsaturated, and polyunsaturated—on blood cholesterol levels revealed that saturated fatty acids tended to raise blood cholesterol levels the most.

It would seem, then, that the *type* of dietary fat, not just fat in general, is specifically related to the risk of developing coronary heart disease, and other chronic diseases. Does this mean some fat is "good" and some fat is "bad"? That we should eat all of one and none of the other?

Actually, the fat issue is a complex one, and not simply a matter of "bad" and "good," as the media often implies. For instance, just because the Cretans drowned their food in olive oil doesn't mean we can do the same and remain slim with unclogged arteries. The residents of rural Crete had far more active lifestyles than most Americans today. Also, scientists now know that fat per se isn't bad. On the contrary, fat is beneficial and even necessary to a healthy, fully functioning body. However, certain types of fat in differing proportions do apparently tend to be more or less beneficial to health.

Americans eat a lot of saturated fat, mostly from animal sources. The residents of Crete during the days of Ancel Keys's research were eating almost all their fat from plant sources, namely olive oil. What's the difference? While oil of any type is 100 percent fat and has the same number of calories as any other oil, each oil or fat type has a different composition—its own ratio of saturated to monounsaturated to polyunsaturated fatty acids. And the fatty acid makeup of an oil appears to make all the difference. The fatty acid composition in, say, a cheeseburger, is far different than the fatty acid composition of a calorie-equivalent portion of olive oil.

Let's look back at Greece. According to Keys, at the time of his research, the general Greek population received approximately 20 percent of their calories from olive oil alone, with total fat intake ranging around 35 percent. (People living on the island of Crete had total fat intakes exceeding 40 percent of daily calories, again, mostly in the form of olive oil, as reported in the *American Journal of Clinical Nutrition*.) Keys describes the rural Greeks, who were accustomed to traditional eating habits and who couldn't afford richer foods, as "remarkably healthy." The wealthier population of Athens, on the other hand, tended to eat food more inspired by the French school of cooking (more prevalent in non-Mediterranean, northern France), which is relatively heavy on butter and crème compared to olive oil. Although no study has proven a direct correlation between these varied diets in Greece and heart disease, Keys could not "help but mention" that Athens had no shortage of wealthy coronary heart disease patients.

Keys's observations significantly complicate the simplified message Americans are accustomed to hearing: that fat is bad and we should eat less of it. Fat is not "bad." We need fat to function. The trick is how to consume it in a way that maximizes our health and gives us the best possible protection against chronic diseases like coronary heart disease and cancer.

❧ WHY WE CRAVE FAT

Long ago, when humans were hunters and gatherers, before we learned to cultivate the land and raise our own food, we relied on our stores of fat to get us through long periods when food was not readily available. To survive, our bodies had to become adept at storing fat. Without it, we would not have survived to today.

Life was hard. Humans had to battle the elements without the luxuries of heating, electricity, and manufactured clothing. We had to hunt for our food instead of buying it at the supermarket. We had to build fires if we wanted to cook our food, and we certainly couldn't drive anywhere. We walked, or ran for our lives, or chased, or climbed, or swam. If we were lucky, once in awhile, we ate to satiety. Life was physically formidable.

Times have changed, of course, especially in America, where food is plentiful for most and automation has largely eliminated the need for physical labor for many people. Although some Americans still squeeze exercise into their days, perhaps a running or jogging session a few times a week or a daily workout at a health club or gym, such a degree of exercise is minimal compared to what humans once were forced to practice. And many Americans don't exercise much at all, spending their days in front of computers or behind counters or in comfortable office chairs.

Yet, no one has informed our bodies that food is now far more accessible than it once was, and that survival requires far fewer calories than it once did. Still lagging behind our rapidly changing industrialized society, our bodies remain genetically engineered to handle prolonged periods without food. We aren't designed for high caloric intakes coupled with low physical activity, yet this scenario describes a way of life for many Americans. The result? An epidemic of obesity, and a high rate of chronic disease. Humans may not die from confrontations with large predatory animals very often anymore, but our lifestyles have evolved in such a way that we are confronted with other perils—heart disease, cancer, diabetes, high blood pressure, and cognitive decline, to name a few.

Our ancient origins also explain why women are more likely to put on excess fat stores during pregnancy, especially during the last trimester. Although women still require extra stores of fat for lactation, our bodies may overzealously prepare, in case of a famine. Long ago, to preserve the survival of the species, women had to be able to provide milk, whether food was roasting on a spit over the fire or not.

Because our bodies remain so proficient at fat storage, to maintain good health and a healthy weight, we must adapt our eating habits to match our twenty-first-century activity levels. Our "antifamine" program tends to convert dietary fat readily into body fat. On the other hand, many researchers believe that carbohydrates are much less readily converted to fat, and are used more easily as ready energy.

What this means is that when we eat too much (as many of us often do), our bodies will convert the excess into body fat. However, some research has shown that if the excess food is carbohydrates rather than dietary fat, the conversion process will take more energy and more time. For people attempting to lose excess weight, reducing calories from dietary fat is a faster way of losing weight than reducing calories from carbohydrates. Of course, all excess calories will eventually be converted to body fat. You can still gain weight eating carbohydrates. Controlled caloric intake is the key to weight loss, but controlled fat-calorie intake makes the job even easier.

Some researchers, such as Dr. Dean Ornish, a medical doctor who has studied the effects of low-fat eating to prevent, control, and even reverse heart disease, believe that almost all fat should be eliminated from the diet, and that only about 10 percent of calories in the diet should come from fat sources. Studies Dr. Ornish has conducted reveal dramatic results in heart disease patients put on a very low-fat diet. However, other researchers believe such a level of dietary fat is too low, especially for those who do not have heart disease, and that a more effective diet substitutes more healthful monounsaturated fats for saturated fats. Such a diet may also be easier to follow, since Americans are so accustomed to a diet higher in fat than Ornish's recommended 10 percent.

One study, "Dietary Oils, Serum Lipoproteins, and Coronary Heart Disease," reported in the *American Journal of Clinical Nutrition*, examined the effects of replacing hard fats in the diet with unsaturated fats such as olive oil, versus the effects of replacing hard fats with carbohydrates. Hard fats are fats that are relatively solid at room temperature and are high in saturated fatty acids or trans fatty acids, such as butter or margarine. Replacing hard fats with unsaturated fats resulted in a more favorable blood cholesterol profile than replacing hard fats with carbohydrates, but only if body weight was kept constant. (The study recognized the danger of obesity from excessive fat consumption.)

But fighting this preprogrammed desire for fat is a challenge. If you are craving a hot fudge sundae or a bag of potato chips, it isn't easy to feel satisfied with a bowl of carrot sticks. You can, however, take comfort in the knowledge that fat cravings often diminish when you get out of the high-fat habit. Once you've become accustomed to the taste of fresh foods unadorned by excess fat—tender vegetables, juicy fruit, wholesome whole grains, and crisp salads like those so celebrated in the traditional Mediterranean cuisines—the taste of too much fat can become unappealing.

✿ FAT TALK

Americans tend to consume about 34 percent of their calories from fat, even though most dietary recommendations suggest we limit fat intake to 30 percent of calories or fewer. More specific recommendations by the American Heart Association (AHA) suggest that fewer than 10 percent of total calories come from saturated fats, 10 to

15 percent from monounsaturated fats, and about 10 percent from polyunsaturated fats. While the average overall fat intake common to the traditional Mediterranean diet is approximately the same as that recommended by the AHA and others, the combinations and proportions of food in the Mediterranean diet suggest that an even lower percentage of saturated fats and a higher percentage of monounsaturated fats might be an even more preferable balance.

In either case, fat is a nutrient required by your body to stay alive. Many experts such as the World Health Organization suggest that *at least* 15 to 20 percent of the total calories you consume should come from fat to keep your body functioning properly.

Fat is a challenge for the weight-conscious, however. With 9 calories per gram (compared to only 4 calories per gram in both carbohydrates and protein), fat packs a caloric punch, and keeping caloric intake under control is important. Obesity (having excessive body fat) increases the risk of many chronic diseases, including heart disease, diabetes, high blood pressure (which further increases the risk of heart disease), and even some cancers. About one third of American adults are obese, and an increasing number of children and adolescents are obese as well.

Yet, the solution to obesity isn't to cut out all fat. As much as our current culture looks askance at body fat (also called adipose tissue), body fat provides stored energy, available for when we need it most. Too much is harmful, but we all need some, and too little fat in the diet can be harmful.

Your body needs some fat for more than energy. Fat helps to keep your skin and hair supple and healthy, helps children to grow properly, insulates your body from temperature extremes, and even protects your internal organs.

Your cell membranes are composed largely of fat. Without fat, your body cannot absorb and deliver vitamins A, D, E, and K. And, while your body makes certain fats, it must derive some from your diet. Two of these are essential: linoleic acid and linolenic acid. (These fats are called "acids" because fatty acids are what make fat.) Eating a variety of foods makes getting enough essential fat in your diet an easy task.

Fat takes longer to digest than other food types, so a meal with a sufficient fat content will generally satisfy your hunger longer than a low-fat meal. It can also make food taste better by adding flavor and texture. Have you noticed that nonfat versions of your favorite foods tend to be less satisfying than the "real thing," even though many low-fat or nonfat foods dramatically boost the sugar content to make up for the lack of "fat flavor"? Consequently, many low-fat and nonfat foods (such as a fat-free Fig Newton cookie) are as high or even higher in calories than the original higher fat version (such as a regular Fig Newton cookie).

However, engaging in a fat free-for-all will make it difficult to remain healthy and at an ideal weight. The point is that fat is necessary, but too much fat can compromise good health. A healthy portion of fat knowhow will help you to include fat in your diet in a way that is beneficial, not destructive, to your health.

✤ FAT IN THE BODY

Fat in the diet has also been linked to an increased risk of heart disease, some cancers, and other chronic diseases. Too much dietary fat can also contribute to obesity, which is a risk factor for a slew of health problems, including coronary heart disease and certain cancers. To understand why too much fat in the diet is dangerous to good health, let's look at what excessive amounts of fat can do in the human body.

A high-fat diet that features the use of foods from animal sources often results in an overconsumption of a particular kind of fat called saturated fat. Too much saturated fat causes blood cholesterol levels to increase, increasing the risk of coronary heart disease. (Blood, or serum, cholesterol refers to the cholesterol in your bloodstream.) Foods high in saturated fatty acids include many types of meat, whole milk, lard, and butter, and a few plant foods such as coconut, palm, and palm kernel oil. Saturated fatty acids may soften at room temperature but still remain relatively firm instead of turning to liquid (like a stick of butter left on the counter—more spreadable but still solid).

Polyunsaturated fatty acids include vegetable oils like corn oil, soybean oil, sunflower oil, and safflower oil, and the fat in most seafood. Polyunsaturated fatty acids are liquid or very soft at room temperature. Some research suggests that excessive amounts of polyunsaturated fatty acids from these vegetable oils are linked to increased risk of cancer, but more research is required to confirm this. In the meantime, polyunsaturated fatty acids in moderate amounts help to keep blood cholesterol levels low because they lower LDL, or "bad," cholesterol levels. They also lower HDL, or "good," cholesterol levels, however, making monounsaturated fatty acids an even better choice.

Monounsaturated fat is the fat type that dominates the traditional Mediterranean diet. Foods rich in monounsaturated fatty acids include olive oil, canola oil, and most nuts and seeds. Liquid at room temperature, monounsaturated fatty acids in the diet have also been shown to lower LDL ("bad") cholesterol levels, but not HDL ("good") cholesterol levels in the blood, making it the fat of choice for a heart-healthy diet.

In other words, what you eat affects the amount of cholesterol in your blood. How much is too much? A serum cholesterol level above 240 mg/dl is considered high, and is associated with an increased risk of coronary heart disease. Between 200 and 239 mg/dl is considered borderline high, and below 200 mg/dl is considered desirable.

Cholesterol levels in the Mediterranean region during the 1960s were generally below 200 mg/dl. Although some of the diets in the traditional Mediterranean region were considered to be high in fat (especially on the isle of Crete), the saturated fat component was low. Because olive oil was the primary source of fat and the use of animal foods was not high, saturated fat intakes were kept in check. Furthermore, with saturated fats low, the heart-healthy monounsaturated fats take center stage.

✬ BLOOD CHOLESTEROL: THE PLAYERS

Your blood cholesterol level can be determined through a simple blood test. Some cholesterol tests give you an overall cholesterol level, and the best tests break down your total cholesterol into LDL and HDL categories. (Those free or low-cost cholesterol screenings you sometimes see at shopping malls tend to give you only overall cholesterol level, while tests performed through your physician are usually more accurate and may give more specific information.)

In general, according to levels set by the National Heart, Lung, and Blood Institute, your total cholesterol level should be under 200 mg/dl, although some researchers, such as Dr. Dean Ornish, feel that a level of 150 mg/dl is more desirable to effectively prevent heart disease. A cholesterol level in the 200 to 239 mg/dl range is a red flag alerting you to be careful and take steps to lower your blood cholesterol. A blood cholesterol level of 240 mg/dl and above puts you at a high risk for heart disease.

Strive to keep your "good" or HDL cholesterol level above 35 mg/dl and your "bad" or LDL cholesterol level below 130 mg/dl. If you haven't had a blood cholesterol test, or if you haven't had one recently, you should be able to schedule a physical exam with your primary care doctor and request a test to determine your blood cholesterol level. Or, if you see one of those free or low-cost tests at your local mall, why not check your blood cholesterol level while it's convenient? If your reading is high, give your physician a call to schedule a more complete test. Blood cholesterol should be screened every five years.

What do the results of a more complete test really mean, and why is "good" cholesterol good and "bad" cholesterol bad? HDL (high-density-lipoprotein) cholesterol is called the "good" cholesterol because this type of cholesterol moves through the body, picks up excess cholesterol, and delivers it to the liver, where it can be eliminated. High levels of HDL cholesterol have been linked to a decreased risk of coronary heart disease. Monounsaturated fats like olive oil have been shown to raise HDL cholesterol levels while lowering levels of LDL. For this reason, monounsaturated fats are recommended to make up the greatest proportion of fats in the diet (as they do in the traditional Mediterranean diet).

LDL (low-density-lipoprotein) cholesterol, the so-called "bad" cholesterol, has been linked to an increased risk of heart disease. LDL cholesterol takes cholesterol from the liver to be deposited throughout the body. (The body needs cholesterol for a variety of purposes, such as making hormones.) Unfortunately, LDL is highly prone to oxidation (more on oxidation later). Oxidized LDL (or o-LDL) is believed to cause damage to the walls of the arteries. Once damaged, fatty deposits (or plaque) can accumulate, which causes the artery walls to harden. Once plaque begins to form, blood is unable to flow as freely. Sometimes so much plaque accumulates that there is a complete occlusion of blood flow. The result is either a heart attack or a stroke.

Once again, saturated fat in the diet has been shown to increase LDL cholesterol levels. Polyunsaturated fats have been shown to lower LDL cholesterol levels, but can also lower HDL cholesterol levels. Best of all, monounsaturated fats like olive oil have been shown to lower LDL cholesterol levels while boosting HDL cholesterol levels.

Keeping LDL blood cholesterol levels low will help to keep our arteries clear, flexible, and healthy, and dietary alterations are among the most effective ways to keep LDL levels in a healthy range.

✣ EATING LESS FAT

One of the best ways to cut fat and saturated fat from your diet is to minimize your consumption of animal products like high-fat meat and dairy products, and maximize your consumption of plant foods. This is the crux of the traditional Mediterranean diet and is easy to visualize with the Mediterranean Diet Pyramid. If plant foods make up the bulk of your diet, you'll need to do little else to keep your saturated fat intake under control.

Center your meals around delicious whole-grain foods and bean dishes, with plenty of vegetables and fruit. Meats and cheeses should be used only as occasional condiments for flavoring. When you fill up on whole grains, vegetables, and fruits, you will not have much room left for high-fat foods.

When you do add fat to your diet, choose a fat rich in monounsaturated fatty acids, like olive oil or canola oil, as often as possible. The alternatives are far less appealing, healthwise. The major sources of saturated fat include butter, shortening, lard, and cocoa butter. These fats should be only on rare occasions, if at all. Olive and canola oil can be used in baking, and there are many ways to avoid the use of saturated fats in traditional American recipes and still produce an excellent dish. Contact the American Dietetic Association (see the Resources section of this book) for recommended cookbooks including such recipes. Coconut, palm, and palm kernel oils are perhaps the most notorious of the plant oils because they are among the few that contain a large proportion of saturated fat (take a deep breath and check the labels of your favorite processed foods).

If most of the fat in your diet comes from monounsaturated fat sources like olive oil and canola oil instead of the many sources of saturated and trans fatty acids fat, you'll find you can indeed eat fat and maintain a healthy heart, as long as you eat fat in moderation, keep your weight at a healthy level, and eat a diet based on plant foods. Remember the Mediterranean Way Pyramid when choosing foods and planning meals. Olive oil is best, but you only need a drizzle, and other high-fat foods should be consumed infrequently.

✽ TRANS FATTY ACIDS AND HYDROGENATION

Trans fatty acids are made from the hydrogenation of unsaturated fats. Recent research has suggested that trans fatty acid, which is found in most margarines, may be as hazardous to our heart health as saturated fats. Confused? Isn't margarine supposed to be better for us than that saturated-fat villain known as butter? This is a question that fuels much debate among nutritionists.

Trans fatty acid is formed when an unsaturated fat, such as polyunsaturated corn oil, is processed in such a way that hydrogen is added into the oil. The result is a more solid fat (making for a better "spread" substitute for butter) and a product that has a longer shelf-life. The drawback? Adding a hydrogen artificially to an otherwise naturally unhydrogenated oil creates a strange chemical formation called "trans." Research has indicated that high levels of these trans fatty acids may increase LDL cholesterol ("bad" cholesterol) levels as much as saturated fat.

So what is a person to do? Do as was done in the traditional Mediterranean cuisine. Use olive oil as your principal form of fat, and limit the use of margarine and butter as much as possible.

Another source of trans fatty acids include prepackaged, processed foods, even most of the "low fat" varieties. Items such as crackers, cookies, chips, granola bars, candy bars, packaged baked goods, even some ready-to-eat cereals and breads contain trans fatty acids. Surprised? That's understandable since, currently, trans fatty acids are almost a hidden ingredient, buried in the long ingredient lists of prepackaged foods. The only way to know if an item has trans fatty acids is to read the label and look for the words *hydrogenated* or *partially hydrogenated oil*. Those words mean trans fatty acids lurk inside. The Food and Drug Administration may soon require that the amount of trans fatty acids be listed on a food product's Nutrition Facts label. For now, however, your best bet is to think "Mediterranean

Way" and minimize these products as much as possible. Fortunately, there are many prepackaged goods that do not contain any trans fatty acids (or hydrogenated or partially hydrogenated oils), but again, read the labels to find which ones are available in your local grocery stores.

ℬ FAT IN THE MEDITERRANEAN

We've already introduced you to the notion that the entire Mediterranean region is olive country and that the primary fat in the Mediterranean diet is olive oil. Olive trees with their fruits burgeoning with oil virtually rim the Mediterranean Sea. When the olives are ripe, they are mashed into a paste and pressed between mats, squeezing the cherished oils into vats below. The process is simple, and the first pressing of the olives yields the olive oil that is the most pure, the most nutrient-rich, and the most flavorful: extra-virgin olive oil. Extra-virgin olive oil is the least processed olive oil.

Depending on the region where the olives were grown, olive oil varies in color, from gold to green. According to Nancy Harmon Jenkins in her *Mediterranean Diet Cookbook*:

> [The] strong-flavored, green-tasting Tuscan oils are very different themselves from the lighter, rounder, fatter oils from Apulia in Italy's South. Which again are distinctive from the oils of Catalonia with their hints of almond and the richer, full-bodied oils from Greece and farther east in Lebanon and the bland, sweet oils from North Africa.

Although strongly (and deliciously) flavored, olive oil is more versatile than some strongly flavored oils because its strong flavor diminishes or disappears when heated. It can, therefore, be used with great success in baking. Lesser grades of olive oil are progressively more processed and refined. Their slightly cheaper prices are not worth the loss of flavor and the benefits of other substances in the oil, not to mention the added undesirable effects of processing. (Keep olive oil out of the light and refrigerate any oil you won't use in one month.)

Although not a component in traditional Mediterranean cuisine, a good olive oil substitute is canola oil, another rich source of monounsaturated fatty acids. Canola oil, sometimes called rapeseed oil, contains a large proportion of monounsaturated fatty acids, like olive oil, as well as vitamin E and omega-3 fatty acids. Although it costs less than its Mediterranean cousin, it is also far more refined and less flavorful. Canola oil is also devoid of phytochemicals (nonnutritive substances in plants that appear to offer protective health effects), those extra "goodies" available in olive oil that has been cold pressed. In terms of a heart-healthy choice, however, it still ranks just below olive oil.

During the time when Ancel Keys was conducting his research, some Mediterranean countries consumed greater or lesser amounts of olive oil. Remember how Cretans were found by Keys to be the olive oil heavyweights, consuming an average of about a half-cup of olive oil per day per person? A full one third of the calories in the Cretan diet came from olive oil. The Greek population in general received about one fifth of its calories from olive oil. Elsewhere throughout the Mediterranean, olive oil consumption was not quite up to Cretan standards, but still far exceeded consumption in the

United States. According to Keys, average olive oil consumption throughout the Mediterranean region equaled about 15 to 20 percent of total calories, "except in the most northerly part of Italy and the non-Mediterranean parts of France and Spain."

Coronary heart disease rates in these countries, as we have mentioned before, were (and still are, although not as dramatically) lower than in the United States, and although olive oil is not the only factor, researchers have narrowed the field enough to surmise that a high proportion of monounsaturated fatty acids in the diet is likely a significant factor in lower coronary heart disease rates.

But olive oil is healthy for more reasons than the monounsaturated fatty acids that lower the risk of coronary heart disease. As mentioned, olive oil contains phytochemicals, more specifically carotenoids, that give vegetables and their oils color, and the antioxidant vitamin E. Antioxidants inhibit the formation of free radicals, elements produced in the body by pollutants and human metabolism that appear to damage the immune system and may contribute to chronic disease. Remember how oxidized LDL leads to hardened and clogged arteries? Vitamin E helps to prevent LDL from oxidizing (antioxidants are explained in more detail in the next chapter).

Again, when it comes to fat, moderation is the key. Focus on consuming a healthy proportion of monounsaturated fats compared to saturated and polyunsaturated fats. Use the Mediterranean Diet Pyramid to help change your diet to reflect the eating patterns and fat consumption of the traditional Mediterranean diet. Overall, fat consumption was moderate, and olive oil was certainly the fat of choice. Olive oil infused the cuisine of the Mediterranean with its rich aroma and its health-bestowing properties. It was (and can still be) a culinary star—but not the only star in a richly varied, heart-healthy, Mediterranean-inspired diet.

✎ RECIPES

The following delicious recipes feature olive oil as a principal ingredient.

✎ TAPENADE

Tapenade is an olive-and-caper paste from the south of France, delicious as an hors d'oeuvre or a light meal spread on French bread, pita wedges, or as a dip for raw vegetables. For a vegetarian option, leave out the tuna.

1½ cups (three 4-ounce cans) ripe olives
¼ cup capers
¼ cup olive oil–packed tuna (or water-packed and well drained—add an additional tablespoon of olive oil)
¼ cup extra-virgin olive oil
2 tablespoons fresh lemon juice
1 tablespoon brandy (optional)
2 cloves garlic, minced

In a blender or food processor fitted with the metal blade, combine all ingredients and process to a chunky paste. Tapenade keeps in the refrigerator for about a week. If the paste is too dry or doesn't blend well, add another tablespoon of olive oil. Serve as a dip for raw vegetables or a spread for fresh bread.

Makes about 2 cups, more or less depending on whether you use the tuna. Enough to serve 6 to 8.

Nutritional Information per ¼-cup serving: 75 calories, 10 grams total fat (7 grams monounsaturated fat, 1 gram polyunsaturated fat, 2 grams saturated fat)

🍃 OLIVE OIL VINAIGRETTE

Americans often select their salad dressings from a prodigious assortment of bottles on the supermarket shelf containing an array of creamy, tangy, or vinaigrette-type dressings in every color and flavor imaginable. In the Mediterranean, the dressing of a salad is a much simpler matter: a little lemon juice or vinegar, some salt and pepper, and a good dose of extra-virgin olive oil. Try mixing up this olive oil vinaigrette at home and you may find it is not only more economical but more delicious and fresh-tasting than bottled dressings.

2 tablespoons balsamic vinegar, good-quality red
    wine vinegar, or fresh lemon juice
1 clove garlic, minced
1 teaspoon salt
Dash of freshly ground black pepper
⅓ cup extra-virgin olive oil

In a small bowl, combine the vinegar or lemon juice, garlic, salt, and pepper. Whisk in the olive oil until well blended. Serve immediately over fresh greens.

Makes just over ¾ cup.

Nutritional Information per tablespoon: 124 calories, 14 grams total fat (10.3 grams monounsaturated fat, 1.2 grams polyunsaturated fat, 1.9 grams saturated fat)

❦ QUESTIONS AND ANSWERS

❦ *How many Americans have high blood cholesterol levels?*

Too many! Approximately half of all Americans have high or borderline-high total blood cholesterol levels. Since blood cholesterol is, in many cases, controllable through dietary changes, you needn't be one of those 50 percent. Try to follow the guidelines of the Mediterranean Way Pyramid to help keep your diet heart-friendly.

❦ *Can blood cholesterol levels be controlled through other methods besides diet?*

Yes. One of the most effective ways to keep total blood cholesterol levels down, as well as increasing "good" or HDL cholesterol levels, is to include lots of physical activity in your life. Exercise can help keep your blood cholesterol profile, as well as your muscles and heart, in great shape. Traditionally the people in the Mediterranean had highly active lifestyles, probably a contributing factor to their excellent heart health.

Smoking has also been linked to increased blood cholesterol levels, so quitting the tobacco habit is an obvious way to help control blood cholesterol levels. Also, obesity tends to raise blood cholesterol, so achieving and maintaining a healthy weight is an effective way for many people to keep blood cholesterol levels in check.

❦ How many Americans die from coronary heart disease?

Too many again. Heart disease is the number one cause of death in America for both men and women. About 25 percent of the 275 million people in America suffer from cardiovascular disease, and over 42 percent of the deaths each year in the United States are due to cardiovascular disease. This includes heart attacks and strokes, both the result of blockages to the blood vessels.

❦ How much fat should I include in my diet?

Your total food choices over the course of a few days should average about 30 percent of calories from fat. But, more importantly, only 10 percent (one third or less of the fat calories) should be from saturated fat. Foods that are high in saturated fat, such as fatty meats, need to be limited as much as possible. Eating in a pattern as described by the Mediterranean Way Pyramid will help to keep saturated fat, as well as total fat and trans fatty acids, within desired levels.

Most packaged food items have the amount of fat and saturated fat grams per serving listed on the Nutrition Facts label. Hopefully, soon the amount of trans fatty acids will be listed as well. If you want to know the percentage of calories from fat and/or saturated fat on any individual food item, you can make the following calculation:

1. Multiply the number of fat or saturated fat grams in a serving by 9 to get the number of calories from fat or saturated fat.
2. Divide the number of calories from fat or saturated fat by the total number of calories per serving.

3. The resulting number is the percentage of calories from fat or saturated fat per serving.

For example, if you want to eat a cup of plain, low-fat yogurt that has 230 calories and 2 grams of fat, multiply 2 grams of fat by 9 to get 18 calories from fat. Then, divide 18 by 230 to get approximately .08, or a total of about 8 percent of calories from fat. To find the amount of saturated fat in the yogurt, look for the grams of saturated fat beneath the total fat grams. If 1 gram of saturated fat is listed, multiply 1 by 9 to get 9 calories from saturated fat. Then, divide by 230 to get approximately .04, or 4 percent of calories from saturated fat—a good choice, especially if you mix in some fresh fruit.

If you wish to calculate the amount of total and saturated fat you eat for any given day, use the following example as a guide. Let's say you require 2,000 calories per day. Then 30 percent of that number is 600 calories; 10 percent is 200 calories. Again, fat has 9 calories per gram, so $600 \div 9 = 67$ grams from total fat, and $200 \div 9 = 22$ grams from saturated fat. Remember, it may be more realistic to think of your fat intake over the course of a few days rather than on a day-to-day basis. You may eat more fat on one day and less on the next, which is fine and in keeping with heart-healthy guidelines.

What about "fat-free" or "low-fat" foods? How do they fit in with a Mediterranean-inspired eating pattern?

Most prepackaged "fat-free" or "low-fat" foods are often high in sugar and/or artificial ingredients, fillers, gums, and other ingredients meant to simulate the taste and texture fat would have provided. These products are often extremely high in calories, lacking in taste, expensive, and devoid of nutrients. In addition, many prepackaged low-fat foods are deceiving because they contain trans fatty acids, which are not listed on the food label. (This will soon be changing as the Food and Drug Administration is considering mandating the amount of trans fatty acids in packaged foods to be listed on food labels.) To eat in a true traditional Mediterranean way, limit the use of these foods as much as possible and opt for foods closer to their natural state. Dried fruit, nuts and seeds, and whole-grain crackers (those without partially hydrogenated oils—read the ingredients) are as convenient to grab on the go as prepackaged snacks. The Mediterranean way of eating is focused on whole, fresh foods.

❧ When eating out, what words suggest lower-fat or higher-fat food preparation?

Lower-fat dishes are often described as baked, broiled, roasted, sautéed, stir-fried, and grilled. Many restaurants will also accommodate your specific cooking suggestions. For example, you may be able to request that olive oil be used in preparing your food, or that your food be cooked with little or no oil. Avoid fried foods and dishes described as creamy, rich, or containing butter- or cream-based sauces, signaling high-fat preparation. Again, remember the Mediterranean Diet Pyramid. Butter, margarine, and high-fat dairy foods sit on the top, which means they are best consumed only on rare occasions.

❧ Olive oil has a strong taste. Is it versatile? How can I replace the fats in my diet with olive oil if I don't care for

the taste, or if the dish I am preparing would not taste good with olive oil?

Olive oil can be an acquired taste, although some people love it upon first try. If you are not immediately charmed, rest assured that in cooking, the strong taste is neutralized. Also, some brands of olive oil taste lighter than others. You can even start with a "light" olive oil, although these are more processed. In general, the lighter in color the olive oil, the lighter in taste. As you get used to the taste of olive oil, you can move on to the darker, richer, more flavorful oils.

If you are not yet used to the taste of olive oil, use it when it will be heated to minimize the taste. In salads and other dishes where oil is not cooked, use canola oil, which is relatively tasteless. You will not receive the same phytochemical benefits, but you will receive the benefits of a monounsaturated fat source. Then gradually introduce olive oil into your diet more often.

Experiment with olive oil in dishes you might not have considered and you may find you are pleasantly surprised at the result. Olive oil in baking imparts a luscious flavor (the baking minimizes the strong olive taste, but leaves just a hint of fruitiness). Pie crusts and other pastries become distinctive with olive oil. Stir a tablespoon into a ho-hum soup to boost its taste and texture. Leave the butter in the refrigerator (or best, at the store) and drizzle a little olive oil on your bread instead. The possibilities are endless.

℘ ***Is it true that oils contain more than one kind of fatty acid?***

Yes. When we say that olive oil is a monounsaturated fat, we mean that it consists primarily of monounsaturated fatty acids. However, olive oil also contains some polyunsaturated fatty acids, and even some saturated fat. Yes, saturated fat, which is why Dr. Dean Ornish, the researcher of low-fat diets to prevent heart disease, promotes such a low-fat diet. All oils contain at least some saturated fat, although in differing amounts. However, the following chart compares a variety of common oils, and as you can see, olive oil and canola oil are the best sources of monounsaturated fat, that type of fat that has been found to increase "good" HDLs and lower "bad" LDLs in the blood.

	Saturated	Mono-unsaturated	Poly-unsaturated
Butter	62%	29%	4%
Canola oil	6%	62%	32%
Coconut oil	87%	6%	2%
Corn oil	13%	24%	59%
Margarine (tub)	14%	32%	31%
Olive oil	14%	77%	8%
Peanut oil	17%	46%	32%
Soybean oil	15%	43%	38%
Sunflower oil	10%	20%	66%

* This chart is adapted from the ADA's complete Food and Nutrition Guide by Roberta Larsun Duyft, Minneapolis: Chronimed, 1996, p. 57

❧ *Is olive oil expensive? How long does it stay fresh? Should it be refrigerated?*

The extra-virgin olive oil on your grocery store shelf is probably the highest quality and least processed of all the oils commonly available, but you will find that a modest bottle often costs quite a bit more than a large bottle of highly refined corn, safflower, sunflower, or canola oil (however, a little olive oil goes a long way). Most oil will last longer if kept in a cool, dark place, preferably in an opaque bottle. The refrigerator is a fine option, and even if it causes your olive oil to congeal or cloud, the oil will return to its clear state when allowed to sit at room temperature. If stored properly, olive oil should last for at least a year. Exposed to light and heat, however, it can quickly turn rancid, like most oils.

❧ *How much olive oil can I eat?*

Olive oil is "drizzled" over the top of our Mediterranean Diet Pyramid to indicate that olive oil should be enjoyed as a highlight to a Mediterranean way of eating, but not to drown out the other healthy benefits. We did not specify actual amounts of oil to be consumed because the amount should really be based on individual calorie needs. Calorie needs are determined from your height, weight, activity level, and state of health. As you can imagine, this can vary greatly from person to person. We strongly suggest consulting with a registered dietitian or other health care provider for guidelines on your individual needs. In general, however, fat should be used in moderation (no need to limit fat intake for children under the age of four, as infants and toddlers need fat for their growth requirements).

And remember how many other spectacular and delicious foods are integral to a traditional Mediterranean diet. Just take a look at the Mediterranean Diet Pyramid if you need a reminder. If too many of the calories in your diet come from olive oil, you won't have room in your calorie allowance for the other good stuff—the whole grains, vegetables, fruits, nuts, beans, and so on—that make up such an important part of a healthy diet.

Olive oil is certainly one of the highlights of the traditional Mediterranean diet and the Mediterranean Diet Pyramid, but it is not the only element. To get maximum health benefits that the traditional Mediterranean diet has to offer, olive oil should be enjoyed in moderation.

4: *Vegetables: The Heart and Soul of the Traditional Mediterranean Diet*

How about a heady minestrone brimming with bright zucchini and carrots, green beans and butternut squash, fragrant garlic and onion, and slivers of plump cabbage leaves for dinner? Or perhaps you would prefer a simple pizza slathered with ruby-red tomato sauce and flecked with fresh basil? Maybe artichoke hearts and tomatoes stuffed with minced onions, cilantro, and a rainbow of chopped bell peppers, Moroccan-style, are more your speed. Chilled tomato-and-pepper gazpacho, anyone? A Greek eggplant salad with red bell peppers, tomatoes, and wild marjoram? Or maybe just a simple antipasti featuring grilled vegetables, marinated olives, and ratatouille?

Fresh and plentiful in the Mediterranean region, vegetables and herbs give traditional Mediterranean cuisine much of its character and flavor, not to mention its beauty and vibrant color. The traditional Mediterranean diet is naturally heavy on vegetables—not surprising, considering the garden-friendly Mediterranean climate. Traditionally many people in the Mediterranean made their living farming the land. Others simply grew food to feed their own families.

What would classic Mediterranean cuisine be without vegetables? From eggplant parmesan and tomatoes Provençal to stuffed vine leaves and spinach-cheese pie, vegetables provide the people of the Mediterranean with variety, color, and flavor without the high cost of meat-based meals. But vegetables, it seems, do much more than provide low-cost meals for people eating them in great quantities in the Mediterranean. Many of the health benefits of the traditional Mediterranean diet are undoubtedly due to the high proportion of fresh vegetables.

There have been many studies that have examined the protective effect of vegetable consumption against certain chronic diseases. Some have uncovered an inverse association between vegetable (and fruit) consumption and the risk of many types of cancers, especially cancers of the upper respiratory and digestive tracts, lungs, stomach, pancreas, and cervix, as well as colorectal and ovarian cancers.

Could vegetable consumption in the Mediterranean be linked to low chronic disease rates? Evidence is mounting to support this theory, even when the evidence doesn't directly involve the Mediterranean. In 1996, researchers Kristi Steinmetz, Ph.D., R.D., and John Potter, M.D., Ph.D., compiled more than two-hundred population and animal studies that looked at plant food consumption and cancer rates. Indeed, there appears to be a strong relationship between plant food consumption and cancer rates. The researchers could only speculate that cancer is a disease resulting from a diet devoid of sufficient amounts of plant foods. Human bodies, it seems, are better able to maintain and even regain their health when plant foods make up the majority of calories in the diet. But that is no surprise to people studying the cuisine and health status of people living in the Mediterranean.

High vegetable consumption seems to have a profound

effect on the occurrence of other chronic diseases, not just cancer. The risk of heart disease, arthritis, macular degeneration (age-associated loss of sight due to gradual degeneration of the macula, a part of the retina), age-related cognitive decline, and other age-related health problems may all be reduced as vegetable consumption increases.

In addition to decreasing the risk of chronic diseases, research suggests that once chronic disease is present, certain components in vegetables may slow or even reverse the progress of the disease. This process occurs perhaps by offering a boost to the immune system, as well as assisting in the fight against cell-damaging free radicals (more on free radicals later in this chapter). In short, research on many fronts strongly suggests that a plant-centered diet rich in vegetables, as well as fruits and whole grains, may add both quality and quantity to your years.

ℬ WHAT MAKES VEGETABLES SO GREAT

Vegetables are more than beautiful and delicious, adding variety and interest to meals. Vegetables are loaded with nutrients such as cancer-fighting folate and selenium, as well as other essential vitamins and minerals. They are also a source of potent phytochemicals such as beta-carotene, lycopene, flavonoids, and thousands of others. Phytochemicals are nonnutritive substances in plants that may serve a variety of protective functions in the human body, from blocking carcinogens and flushing them out of the body to strengthening the immune system (more on phytochemicals later in this chapter).

Vegetables are also low in calories, making this the food group in which you can really indulge. On top of all these benefits, vegetables are rich in fiber, which has been linked to decreased cancer risk and also helps to fill you up and keep your digestive tract working smoothly.

Every vegetable is its own unique package of nutrients and phytochemicals, so to reap the most benefit, eat a wide variety of vegetables. Remember the Mediterranean Diet Pyramid, not to mention the USDA's emphasis on variety? Vegetables are the perfect food group with which to follow these guidelines. Their great variety and range of flavors, textures, and colors make them the perfect food group around which to base a meal.

Remember to sample vegetables from all of the following categories. A handful of veggies from each category thrown into a soup pot with some chicken stock or vegetable stock and some dried oregano, fresh basil or thyme leaves, and a clove or two of minced garlic makes a fantastic, Mediterranean-inspired vegetable soup!

- **Cruciferous Vegetables.** These vegetables, which include broccoli, Brussels sprouts, cabbage, bok choy, cauliflower, kale, kohlrabi, and greens like watercress, mustard, rutabaga, and turnip, are so named because their flower petals are arranged in a cross shape (*crucifer* means "cross-bearing"). Even though not all of these mentioned vegetables are native to the Mediterranean regions (such as bok choy), they can and should be eaten in a Mediterranean-inspired diet. Cruciferous vegetables are acclaimed for their health effects, and none more so than broccoli, a nutritional "star" rich with fiber, vitamins A and C, folate, calcium, iron, potassium, magnesium, and a host of phytochemicals including beta-carotene found to be active in the human body. Many cruciferous vegetables are already featured in traditional Mediterranean dishes: cabbage in minestrone soup or boiled and then baked with olive oil and garlic; steamed broccoli with garlic, olive oil, and hot peppers or cooked until tender and tossed with a variety of pasta shapes; Brussels sprouts in a white sauce with a little grated cheese, nutmeg, and pine nuts; kale tossed with chestnuts, onion, and a little bacon.

- **Solanacae Vegetables.** This family of vegetables includes the tomato, pepper, potato, and eggplant. These vegetables are good sources of vitamins A and C and potassium. Tomatoes have recently been in the spotlight because of a phytochemical called lycopene that gives them (as well as watermelons and red grapefruit) their red color. Lycopene is particularly concentrated in tomato sauce and tomato paste, and research has linked high lycopene consumption with reduced risk of prostate cancer and some other cancers. The solanacae family of vegetables is heavily featured in traditional Mediterranean dishes. What would Italian cuisine be without the tomato? A simple sauce of ripe, fresh crushed tomatoes and a little olive oil is all a good pasta really needs. (Because lycopene is fat-soluble, it becomes even more available to the body when tomatoes are cooked in a small amount of oil). When tomatoes are combined with eggplant in fragrant dishes such as ratatouille or eggplant Parmesan, these vegetables are a mouthwatering treat. Other favorite dishes include peppers roasted with eggplant; potatoes boiled with garlic cloves and mashed together; baba ghanouj, an eggplant dip popular in the Middle East; and any or all of these vegetables roasted, sautéed, or lightly boiled and tossed with pasta, rice, polenta, or eaten on their own.

- **Umbelliferous Vegetables.** These vegetables have umbrella-like leaves. They include carrots, celery, parsnips, fennel, and the herbs parsley and cilantro. Umbelliferous vegetables are rich in beta-carotene, vitamin A, and vitamin C. Although not used as heavily in traditional Mediterranean cuisine as vegetables such as eggplant and tomatoes, umbelliferous vegetables are certainly present in farmer's markets and on the table. Parsley and cilantro are featured herbs in many traditional Mediterranean dishes. According to Nancy Harmon Jenkins in her *Mediterranean Diet Cookbook*, Italians use raw fennel to cleanse the palate after a meal and often serve it sliced and sprinkled with olive oil and lemon juice. Carrots are featured in many different salads in the Middle East, paired with fruit or cheese or yogurt, and also in soups and stews in virtually every Mediterranean country. Both carrots and celery are standard ingredients in an Italian minestrone soup, and Ancel Keys's book *How to Eat Well and Stay Well the Mediterranean Way* contains a recipe for braised celery and carrots, called céleri et carottes Provençale in France and sedano e carota in Italy.

- **Cucurbitaceous Vegetables.** Offerings from this family of vegetables include the gourds and melons, those fleshy fruits and vegetables that grow on vines. These include pumpkins, summer squash, winter squash, zucchini, cucumbers, honeydew melons, and watermelons. Cucurbitaceous vegetables are rich sources of vitamins A and C, beta-carotene, phosphorous, iron, and fiber. While squash isn't typically considered a part of traditional Mediterranean cuisine, zucchini is the one exception. Ubiquitous in many Italian soups and stews as well as stuffed, grilled, baked, stewed, mixed with pasta, tossed into an Italian frittata, or cooked with tomatoes for ratatouille, zucchini is an Italian favorite.

- **Allium Vegetables.** These vegetables (some are considered herbs) include those Mediterranean staples, garlic and onions. They also include shallots, chives, and leeks. Allium vegetables are thought to contain a host of cancer-fighting phytochemicals, and may also have antibiotic properties. Flip through any Mediterranean-inspired cookbook and you'll see garlic and, slightly less frequently, onions featured in just about every recipe that isn't a dessert. Garlic is also fantastic and surprisingly mellow as the featured ingredient in a Spanish garlic soup. Who can forget the rich aroma and savory taste of French onion soup brimming with tender sweet onions, flavored with a splash of brandy, and topped with a slice of French bread and a little grated cheese? According to Ancel Keys, the Italian version of liver and onions is far heavier on the onions than on the liver, and stifado, a Greek beef stew, contains more onions than beef.

✼ VEGETABLE TALK

Nowhere are vitamins, minerals, and phytochemicals more densely concentrated than in vegetables. If you do not typically include a lot of vegetables in your diet, knowing a little more about the health-boosting elements in vegetables may inspire you to increase your vegetable consumption. Let's start with vitamins.

� VITAMINS

Vitamins are chemical substances in vegetables (and other foods) that have a variety of jobs in the body, from assisting the chemical reactions that make your body function to promoting growth to preventing infection. There are two kinds of vitamins: water soluble and fat soluble.

Water-soluble vitamins dissolve in water and are carried through your bloodstream quickly. These vitamins, which include thiamin, riboflavin, niacin, vitamin B_6, folacin, vitamin B_{12}, biotin, pantothenic acid, and vitamin C, must be ingested regularly because the body doesn't store them. Among the many life-supporting functions of water-soluble vitamins, folacin and vitamin C have been shown to have anticancer functions, especially when paired with the fat-soluble vitamin E and beta-carotene (a form of vitamin A).

The fat-soluble vitamins—A, D, E, and K—dissolve in fat and are stored in your body for longer periods of time. (For example, the body is capable of storing up to a year's supply of vitamin A alone!) Beta-carotene (a form of vitamin A found in vegetables) and vitamin E have been given a lot of attention lately as powerful antioxidants (more on antioxidants later). Many studies have linked these nutrients with the prevention of certain chronic diseases such as cancer and heart disease. Although the major food sources of vitamin E are nuts (especially the almond), seeds (especially sunflower seeds), wheat germ, and certain oils, there are a few vegetables that also contain appreciable amounts of vitamin E, most notably the sweet potato and avocado. Because many vegetables contain vitamin A, we will highlight this powerful nutrient (along with the other cancer-fighting vitamins, C and folacin) below.

In keeping with the spirit of the traditional Mediterranean diet, we recommend getting your vitamins from vegetables (and the other foods listed in the "daily" and "weekly" sections of the Mediterranean Diet Pyramid) rather than from supplements. Nutritional supplements were unheard-of in traditional Mediterranean culture, and were most likely not needed given the nutrient density of the diet. We suggest getting your vitamins and other nutrients the way nature intended!

Vitamin A

Famous for promoting good vision, this fat-soluble vitamin is involved in a number of other important bodily processes. Vitamin A plays a vital role in maintaining healthy skin and healthy tissues found in your mouth, genitals, and digestive and urinary tracts. It also assists with the proper development of fetuses, sperm production, growth of children, and more. In terms of cancer prevention, vitamin A's importance in supporting the immune system makes this nutrient a powerful ally in the fight against cancer.

Getting adequate amounts of vitamin A is easy in a vegetable-rich Mediterranean diet. Vegetable sources that contain vitamin A are easy to identify. Just look for the color orange, and you've got beta-carotene—a form of vitamin A. Beta-carotene, a phytochemical that we'll discuss below, is a potent antioxidant. Sweet potatoes, carrots, and melons are common traditional Mediterranean foods and they are excellent sources of beta-carotene.

Pumpkin, although a native North American vegetable, is another rich source of beta-carotene and can easily be included in a Mediterranean diet.

Vitamin C

Vitamin C, also called ascorbic acid, was first made famous for warding off scurvy in sailors long ago. Scurvy, a condition that is characterized by swollen, bleeding gums and tooth loss, is rarely seen today, usually only in the very malnourished. Vitamin C's next claim to fame has been its apparent ability to fight off the common cold. Because of this potential cold-busting capacity, many Americans have become accustomed to loading up on vitamin C supplements, but how much vitamin C is actually needed to help ward off the common cold is still unknown. What *is* known is that taking large doses of this vitamin can lead to more serious problems, such as the formation of kidney stones and diarrhea. Vitamin C is also known for its ability to help the body absorb the iron found in plant foods. So, the vitamin C–rich Mediterranean Way diet helps to insure adequate iron absorption for the average adult.

Recently, this vitamin has become associated with chronic disease prevention, namely heart disease and cancer. Vitamin C's antioxidant abilities and its important role in maintaining a strong immune system is one reason, but its other role of collagen production makes vitamin C all the more beneficial in cancer prevention. Collagen is a protein-based substance that acts as structural material in skin, muscle, lung, and bone. The stronger this structural material, from a diet rich in vitamin C, the less likely cancer will invade these tissues. The presence of vitamin C in the digestive tract has been shown to prevent the formation of nitrosamines, those believed cancer-causing substances found in cured meats.

Vitamin C also works hand in hand with vitamin E to deactivate cancer-promoting free radicals.

In addition to cancer prevention, vitamin C helps to promote a healthy heart. There is even some evidence that increased intake of vitamin C may help to improve one's blood cholesterol profile by lowering the level of "bad" LDLs and raising the level of "good" HDLs.

The recommended daily allowance (RDA) of vitamin C for the average adult is 60 milligrams. Pregnant women need 70 milligrams and breast-feeding moms need about 90 to 95 milligrams per day. Many researchers feel that more than this is needed to prevent disease, although just how much is still unknown. Smokers do need to get more than the standard RDA, about 100 milligrams daily, because smoking can deplete the body of this nutrient. Getting adequate amounts of vitamin C can easily be done in a varied Mediterranean-type diet that is rich in fruits and vegetables. Eat just one orange, and you've already consumed 60 milligrams of vitamin C. Many vegetables are also rich sources of vitamin C. Those most relevant to the traditional cuisine of the Mediterranean include tomatoes, green and red peppers, broccoli, spinach, potatoes, and asparagus.

Folacin

The word *folacin* is from the Latin word *folium*, or "foliage," because folic acid was first discovered in leafy green vegetables. Also known as folate or folic acid, this water-soluble B vitamin is essential for several important functions in the body. For one, it is crucial in the synthesis of DNA, and because of this, any body tissue that is dividing and growing needs ample amounts of folacin. Cells lining our digestive tract are continually regenerating themselves and therefore rely on folacin to do so.

Pregnant women need substantial amounts of folate (more than twice the RDA for the average adult) to support the growing fetus. The U.S. Public Health Service recommends that all women of childbearing age eat 400 micrograms of folacin daily to ensure adequate stores of folacin to support the large demands of this nutrient in pregnancy. Women who enter into pregnancy without adequate folacin stores and/or those who do not eat enough folacin during pregnancy (particularly in the first trimester) run the risk of bearing a baby with inadequate brain and spinal cord development.

Folacin's supporting role in DNA synthesis appears to make this nutrient important in the battle against cancer, particularly cancer of the colon. In 1993, the *Journal of the National Cancer Institute* reported that "those eating more folate rich foods are less likely to develop colon cancer." Some researchers feel that intakes of 400 to 800 micrograms of folacin are needed for cancer prevention, but this is still being determined. The Mediterranean Way diet provides ample amounts of folacin, especially with its emphasis on bean and vegetable consumption (see the following Q & A section). The vegetables that are richest in folacin include avocados, artichokes, asparagus, spinach, mustard spinach (tendergreen), and turnip greens. These vegetables were highly celebrated in most traditional Mediterranean cooking.

❧ THE POWER OF ANTIOXIDANTS

Antioxidants are substances that combat the negative effects of oxygen in cells. When the body uses oxygen for energy, it produces by-products called free radicals that have a potentially damaging effect on cells. Antioxidants neutralize this effect, essentially shuttling free radicals and even carcinogenic substances out of the body before they can do damage.

Three of the most potent antioxidants are the vitamins C, E, and the substance beta-carotene, which the body converts to vitamin A. These vitamins have been a long-time research focus in disease prevention, and have been repeatedly linked to decreased risk of many chronic conditions, including heart disease, cancer, cataracts, and more. Research with the AIDS virus suggests that vitamin E and beta-carotene may slow the progression of HIV to AIDS. Vitamin E is thought to protect from heart disease in a number of ways, by slowing or preventing oxidation of "bad" (LDL) cholesterol, and possibly by reducing the tendency of blood to clot.

The protective antioxidant power of vitamin E has also been shown to increase dramatically when vitamin C and beta-carotene are also consumed. Shown to work in concert to modify the risk of many chronic diseases and age-related degenerative conditions, a balance of these three antioxidants seems to be most effective in the body, and the absence of one seems to negatively impact the effectiveness of the others. For example, vitamin C flushes out free radicals in the body's fluids, while beta-carotene and vitamin E neutralize free radicals in fat tissue.

Not long ago, beta-carotene was shown to be a gold star in the world of cancer prevention, and supplementation with this nutrient became popular. It seemed to make sense, given its antioxidant capabilities. However, recent research using beta-carotene supplements brought about some surprising results. In one famous study, beta-carotene supplementation was linked with an *increase* (not a decrease) in lung cancer among subjects that smoked. (This is an example of the possible dangers of supplementation.) Study subjects who did not smoke, however, were not negatively affected by the supplementation. Smokers typically have depleted stores of vitamins C as well as E.

Of course, no such toxicity has been shown to exist when beta-carotene is consumed via vegetables. On the contrary, studies suggest that vitamins from food sources have a positive effect on a number of chronic conditions. One study linked increased vitamin C and beta-carotene consumption primarily from food (as opposed to supplements) to better old-age memory in a long-term Swiss study begun in 1971 and published in 1997.

However, the results of studies seeking to determine the value of vitamin supplements are, in general, hazy. Some research seems to suggest supplements can have a positive effect on health (especially with vitamin E). Other studies suggest supplements have no effect. Still others indicate that vitamin supplements, especially in megadoses, can actually be injurious to health. However, vitamins in their natural form—potently supplied in vegetables—appear to be beneficial to health in countless, complex ways, as yet only minimally understood.

Just about every vegetable is packed with vitamins, and the traditional Mediterranean diet supplies vitamin-rich vegetables in abundance, and in far higher proportion than is typical in the American diet. Eating more vegetables, and a wider variety of vegetables, is an excellent first step toward eating in a Mediterranean-inspired fashion. It is also the safest and probably most effective way to reap the benefits of the many vitamins—antioxidants and others—your body requires.

❧ MUST-HAVE MINERALS

Minerals work with vitamins in many bodily processes, and regulate a few essential functions, such as muscle contractions and nerve impulses. They are also part of our bodies: bones, teeth, and nails all contain minerals. The major minerals, including calcium, magnesium, and potassium, can all be found in certain vegetables. Many vegetables contain trace minerals as well, such as iron, selenium, and zinc.

Selenium has been the subject of much research. Another antioxidant, selenium appears to boost the action of certain anticancer enzymes in the body, and may even prevent premature aging. Plants incorporate selenium from the soil in which they are grown. Garlic is a good source of selenium.

Calcium is essential for bone strength and to slow the rate of bone loss associated with aging. Calcium also assists muscle contractions, including the heart muscle; facilitates proper nerve functioning; and helps the blood to clot. Calcium deficiencies can result in osteoporosis and may contribute to high blood pressure and possibly colon cancer. While most people think of dairy products as the best sources of calcium (they are indeed good sources of calcium), many vegetables supply calcium as well. In fact, the calcium in some vegetables (such as kale) is even more available to the body than the calcium in dairy products. Other calcium-rich vegetables include dark leafy greens such as mustard greens, turnip greens, and broccoli.

Magnesium is another mineral essential to bone strength and growth, as well as in nerve and muscle cells. It warrants a mention here because magnesium and calcium work together in the body to perform many important functions, and a magnesium deficiency also hinders the body's ability to use calcium (as well as potassium and sodium). Rich sources include dark green vegetables like spinach, as well as other foods common to the Mediterranean diet such as whole grains, nuts, and legumes.

ℬ PHYTOCHEMICALS: NATURE'S FIRST LINE OF DEFENSE

The buzz about vitamins and minerals has lately been replaced by the buzz about phytochemicals. Phytochemicals are nonnutritive substances in plants. Thousands exist, and every plant food contains them. What can they do for us? Knowing what they do for plants may shed some light on the question.

Some phytochemicals protect plants from invaders of all kinds. Predators like leaf-munching insects and animals, bacteria, viruses, and fungi can all be put off by the action of phytochemicals, whether that action comes in the form of an unpleasant taste, a repugnant smell, a startling color, or a poisonous effect. Also, the antioxidant action of certain phytochemicals protects plants against an oxygen-rich environment (remember, plants "breathe" carbon dioxide, not oxygen).

What happens when we consume phytochemical-laden vegetables? Only some of the thousands of phytochemicals have been found (to date) to have an effect on the human body, but these few apparently have enough of an effect to make a difference. (The thousands of phytochemicals as yet unresearched represent great research potential. The field of phytochemical research is still in its infancy and may well reveal myriad other benefits to human health.)

When humans consume certain phytochemicals, we appear to enjoy protective effects similar to those plants receive. Phytochemicals, in many ways, seem to defend the human body against free radical damage (see below) and age-related degeneration, not to mention viruses, bacteria, and fungi.

The phytochemical-cancer connection has been widely

researched, and results suggest that phytochemicals may disrupt cancer in more ways than one. Phytochemicals may protect DNA or repair damaged DNA, helping to prevent cancer from developing. They may prevent cancerous cells from multiplying and/or spreading through the body. Phytochemicals may help the body to help itself, giving carcinogen-blocking enzymes a boost.

Much cancer research has focused more generally on vegetable and fruit consumption, which implicates phytochemicals by association. Raw and green vegetable consumption appears to reduce the risk of stomach, lung, mouth, esophageal, colon, rectal, breast, and bladder cancers. Research in other areas has supported general vegetable and fruit consumption as well, suggesting that a diet rich in vegetables and fruits may lower the risk of heart disease and stroke, and boost the effectiveness of the immune system.

Some of the phytochemicals more relevant to humans include the allium compounds (in onions and garlic); carotenoids (in dark green and deep orange vegetables), including lycopene (particularly rich in tomatoes and red grapefruit); glucosinolates (in cruciferous vegetables such as broccoli); and flavonoids (in many foods including tomatoes).

Aromatic Allium

Allium compounds, also called organosulfides, exist in onions, garlic, leeks, shallots, and chives. These compounds give these vegetables their unique smell and pungent taste. They also appear to increase the effectiveness of the body's own cancer-fighting enzymes, halt the production of nitrates into carcinogens, lower cholesterol and blood pressure, and reduce the tendency of the blood to clot. Allium compounds appear to be most potent in raw vegetables, and may be destroyed by the cooking process.

Colorful Carotenoids

Carotenoids are potent antioxidant phytochemicals that fight free-radical cellular damage in the body, possibly guarding against a wide range of chronic diseases. They are the substances in plants that provide their bright red, orange, or deep yellow colors. More than six hundred carotenoids are known, but fewer than fifty have been found to be active in the human body. Examples of beneficial carotenoids found in vegetables are as follows:

- Alpha-carotene, which the body converts to vitamin A. Research has linked alpha-carotene to a reduced risk of lung cancer. Carrots are full of it.
- Beta-carotene (as discussed previously) is another substance the body converts to vitamin A. Well publicized for its anticancer benefits, beta-carotene may also prevent cataracts, slow the progression of heart disease, and boost the immune system. Good sources include most red, orange, and yellow fruits and vegetables, as well as dark, leafy greens. A recent famous study showed that beta-carotene supplements actually increased the risk of lung cancer in study subjects who smoked, but no such link has been found with the nonsmoking study participants. Nevertheless, because so little is known about phytochemicals, we recommend reaping their benefits from food sources, not from supplements.
- Gamma-carotene is just starting to get attention as an anticancer agent, and research with gamma-carotene is just beginning. The best sources of gamma-carotene are tomatoes and apricots. The above three carotenoids—alpha-

carotene, beta-carotene, and gamma-carotene, are thought to be powerful allies against cancer.

- Lycopene, the carotenoid that gives tomatoes, watermelon, and red grapefruit their rosy hues, has been linked to decreased risk of prostate and breast cancer, and may also protect skin from the damaging effects of ultraviolet radiation.
- Lutein and zeaxanthin have been found in the eye and may help prevent age-related macular degeneration by protecting the retina from potentially harmful light exposure, and also by neutralizing the effects of free radicals formed by the negative effects of sunlight on the retina. One study demonstrated a lower incidence of macular degeneration in people who ate increased amounts of spinach and collard greens, both of which contain lutein and zeaxanthin.

✌ PROTECTIVE FLAVONOIDS

Flavonoids include a huge class of compounds (more than four thousand) called phenolic compounds and are found in plants of all types. Flavonoids give plants color, have antifungal properties, slow or prevent damaging oxidation, lower cholesterol, prevent the clotting of blood, and protect cells from carcinogens. The most studied flavonoid is quercetin, abundant in onions, wine, and tea (more on wine in the next chapter). Unlike the allium compounds, quercetin remains intact and available after cooking, and may have an anticancer effect in the body.

Other flavonoids available to the human body from food include isoflavones, found primarily in soybeans (although soybeans aren't part of a traditional Mediterranean diet, their health benefits warrant a mention). Isoflavones are thought to have an estrogen-like effect on the body, possibly guarding against hormone-related cancers like breast cancer. Catechins are another type of flavonoid, which may be responsible for the anticancer properties apparently inherent in green tea. Flavonoids may also be a factor in the heart-protective benefits of red wine.

☙ PHYTOCHEMICAL SYNERGY

One of the most intriguing qualities of phytochemicals, and the most convincing argument for receiving your phytochemicals from food rather from supplements, is their synergistic nature. Science has only begun to understand the effects of individual phytochemicals on the body. The combined nature of phytochemical interactions in the body—of eating a whole plant, rather than a supplement of artificially produced or isolated single compound—is still largely a matter of speculation, but many experts assert that eating plant foods in a form close to their original state (minimally processed) is the best way to ensure receiving the health benefits, both those understood and not yet understood.

Even if the term *phytochemical* was unknown in the Mediterranean during the time when the traditional Mediterranean diet was the pervasive way of eating, phytochemical benefits were at a premium in this diet of locally grown, seasonally consumed, minimally processed plant foods. Understanding the nature of phytochemicals provides one more good reason to return to more traditional dietary practices.

❦ FREE RADICALS, OXIDATION, AND ANTIOXIDANTS: SUMMON YOUR DEFENSES

Vitamins C, E, and beta-carotene aren't the only antioxidants. Many phytochemicals also have antioxidant properties, from which we derive great benefit. *Antioxidant*, once again, is a term referring to any substance that helps to nullify the deleterious, albeit natural, side effects of oxygen consumption within cells. Oxygen may seem like a harmless substance. We breathe it in all day long. All cells require oxygen to function. Oxygen is necessary for human life. However, oxygen consumption releases by-products that are potentially damaging to cells.

In our bodies, when cells use oxygen for energy, they produce by-products or waste products called free radicals. Free radicals are oxygen by-products missing an electron, which they have given up during the oxidation process. Free radicals "roam" through the body searching for electrons to correct the imbalance. The nearest molecule with an available electron is "robbed" by the free radical, and every cell robbed of an electron is slightly damaged. This is a natural process. Our cell membranes contain vitamin E to help neutralize free radical activity before cell damage can occur. However, our bodies weren't designed to handle the onslaught of free radicals produced by environmental pollutants common to everyday life today: car exhaust, cigarette smoke, and so on. Without sufficient antioxidant protection, over time, free radical damage can become an insurmountable obstacle to good health. Many scientists believe that cumulative free radical damage contributes to chronic diseases like cancer, heart disease, arthritis, and macular degeneration.

The name *antioxidant* suggests that these compounds

nullify the negative effects of oxidation on cells, and that is exactly what they do. If you dipped a cut piece of apple in lemon juice, it wouldn't turn brown as quickly because lemon juice contains ascorbic acid (a common form of vitamin C), an antioxidant. Another form of oxidation occurs when fat turns rancid. Tocopherols, a common form of vitamin E, are often used to preserve foods with fat because the vitamin E retards the oxidation, or spoilage, process.

Exactly how antioxidants work is still largely unknown, but antioxidants appear to work in several ways in the body. Antioxidants seem to prevent free radical damage in the first place. They also may shuttle carcinogenic compounds generated by free radical damage out of the body before they can do any damage. And, as we've mentioned before, while the verdict is not yet in on whether antioxidant vitamin supplements do any good at all in the prevention of chronic disease, antioxidant consumption from fresh vegetables does seem to offer a significant measure of protection against free radical damage.

✿ MEDITERRANEAN WAYS TO ADD VEGETABLES

How did the people eating the traditional Mediterranean diet pack so many vegetables into their daily meals? Easily and deliciously. In the Mediterranean, vegetable consumption is not just a matter of eating any vegetable at any time, in whatever state is most convenient. Vegetable selection is a matter of pride, vegetable preparation an art, and vegetable consumption a pure pleasure. Most essentially, in the Mediterranean, vegetables are chosen according to what is in season.

Outdoor produce markets throughout the Mediterranean offer the season's best, freshest, most vibrant vegetables. Your local grocer, farmer's market, or produce stand is also likely to feature the freshest locally grown produce. Even if the vegetables in season in your area aren't those in season in the Mediterranean, eating the freshest seasonal produce is still eating in the Mediterranean way. Seek out excellent sources for vegetables in your area (more difficult in some areas during some seasons) and you may discover that vegetables taste much better than you remember.

Here are a few more Mediterranean-inspired tips for adding vegetables to your day. You'll wonder how you ever ate without them!

- Looking for a fast-food lunch? A wedge of hearty wheat bread, a small chunk of feta or other cheese, a few slices of ripe tomato, a handful of leafy greens drizzled with olive oil and a squeeze of fresh lemon juice, and a ripe peach or other seasonal fruit for dessert take less time to prepare than going through the drive-through. Bring your Mediterranean lunch to work with you and everyone will wonder what upscale deli supplied your meal.
- The next time you make spaghetti, stir a shredded carrot and a finely chopped green or red pepper, a few mushrooms, or a handful of chopped spinach into the sauce. Vegetable additions add color, flavor, and nutritional power to your pasta dinner.
- Instead of grilling burgers, grill vegetables, Mediterranean style. Slice onions, peppers, zucchini, large mushrooms, eggplant, and tomatoes into thick slices, drizzle with olive oil, and grill. If you want to add a Middle Eastern flair, skewer

the vegetables into shish kebabs. A chunk or two of chicken or lamb among the vegetables would be authentic and would add an extra dash of protein. Serve with lemon wedges.

• Drizzle those plain vegetables with a little olive oil and a sprinkling of fresh grated cheese, or garnish with a splash of tomato sauce or a few sun-dried tomatoes. Tomato sauce also adds culinary interest to broiled fish.

• If you can relate to former U.S. President George Bush when it comes to broccoli (his aversion to this beautiful vegetable was well known), maybe you just haven't had it cooked really well. Try steaming broccoli just until it is very bright green and tender. Toss with a little olive oil, salt, minced garlic, and a few flakes of red pepper. Serve and eat immediately. Perfectly cooked broccoli is a joy. Overcooked or old broccoli is enough to make anyone dislike the stuff.

• Leafy green salads are an important part of many Mediterranean meals. Get in the habit of including a bowl of leafy greens with olive oil and a little lemon juice or vinegar with at least one meal every day. A few extra chopped vegetables and a little grated cheese will make your greens even more interesting and nutrient-rich. (Just remember to forego the creamy dressing in favor of a dressing with an olive oil base.) Do you think you don't have enough time to chop up a salad? Take advantage of food industry technology and splurge on ready-to-eat bagged veggies and greens. Selections are plentiful, many types are organic, and they come prewashed.

• Eat pizza in the Mediterranean style. Unlike American pizzas, Mediterranean pizzas are typically thin, light concoctions with just a few toppings. Fresh tomato sauce and one or two featured vegetables (mushrooms, garlic slices, onion, zucchini, broccoli, peppers) and a very light sprinkling of mozzarella cheese on a fresh-baked (or store-bought, if you are pressed for time) whole-grain crust makes a perfect light dinner. In the mood for something more substantial? The more veggies, the better! Add roasted eggplant, mushrooms, red peppers (better than green if you want that lycopene punch)—you name it! See how much your pizza can hold. Load up and enjoy!

- Are you or your kids getting bored with peanut butter sandwiches? Add chopped or shredded carrots for a surprising, refreshing, flavorful crunch.

- Pumpkin is an American vegetable, but its nutritional value is Mediterranean in spirit! Stir canned pumpkin into hot oatmeal for breakfast with a little cinnamon and brown sugar. Add a generous spoonful to applesauce for a light dessert, or stir some into vanilla yogurt for an added zing.

- Microwave a sweet potato or yam until soft for a quick, carotenoid- and fiber-rich snack, or try baked sweet potato fries or yam chips, brushed lightly with olive oil and baked at 400 degrees until lightly browned and fork-tender, about twenty minutes, or longer if you've got a large pan full.

The one thing you can do to make your diet more "Mediterranean" is to begin eating more fresh vegetables today. Whether or not they were traditionally grown and consumed in the Mediterranean, the very concept of eating the vegetables grown on the land around you captures the essence of the traditional Mediterranean diet. Vegetables add beauty to your plate, excitement to your palate, and a host of vital substances to your body.

☙ QUESTIONS AND ANSWERS

☙ *If allium compounds are destroyed in the cooking process, what is the best way to include them in the diet? Raw onions and garlic?*

To many people, raw onions and garlic are too strongly flavored to be palatable when eaten alone. However, minced or even thinly sliced raw onions are an aromatic addition to a salad, and minced fresh garlic tastes great in an olive oil vinaigrette salad dressing. Raw chives are another delicious addition to salads and make a crunchy garnish to other foods, from the traditional cottage cheese to grain-based dishes and pasta dishes. When you do cook onions and garlic, try to cook them for as short a time as possible. When making soups and stews, sprinkle a few chopped onions on top, and/or add the garlic (or half the garlic) toward the end of the cooking time.

☙ *Are the familiar herbs and spices used in Mediterranean cuisine of any nutritional value, or are they purely for flavoring?*

Herbs and spices are plant foods and are rich with nutrients and phytochemicals, just like vegetables, although research hasn't focused its attention on herbs and spices the way it has on vegetables (at least partially due to the fact that these plant foods are consumed in much smaller amounts and so may have a less potent, although quite possibly cumulative, effect). Some plant foods such as garlic are often thought to be either an herb or a vegetable, and the distinction is indeed blurry at times. The dictionary even defines vegetables as "a usually herbaceous plant cultivated for its edible parts." Herbs are, technically, plants with fleshy rather than woody stems, and are also defined as "aromatic plants used in medicine or as seasoning." Similarly, spices are "aromatic or pungent plant substances used as flavoring."

While different Mediterranean countries tend to emphasize different herbs and spices, the region as a whole seems particularly partial to the following, listed below along with their nutritive and/or phytochemical highlights:

- **Garlic and chives.** Members of the allium family, these herbs contain organosulfides, the compounds that give allium vegetables their unique odors. Organosulfides are thought to have anticancer properties and to benefit heart health. Garlic also contains phenolic acids, antioxidant compounds that may disrupt cancer development in several ways, and monoterpenes, substances that appear to slow or reverse cancer development and contribute to favorable blood cholesterol profiles. Chives contain the carotenoids lutein and zeaxanthin, antioxidants that concentrate in the eye. Dried or dehydrated chives provide an even more concentrated source of these phytochemicals. Garlic is highly versatile and can flavor almost any savory dish. Sprinkle chopped chives, fresh or dried, on eggs, fish, or a salad.

- **The rosemary family of herbs.** Oregano, basil, thyme, marjoram, sage, mint, and rosemary are all members of the Labitaceae family and all contain the powerful antioxidant quinone. Oregano, basil, and thyme are pervasive in Mediterranean, especially Italian, cuisine, and give dishes like pizza, spaghetti, and lasagna their familiar flavors.

- **Parsley and cilantro.** These members of the umbelliferous family of vegetables (related to the carrot) are nutritional power herbs. The most widely used herb in the United States today, parsley dates back to the third century B.C. and was popular among the Romans. Parsley can be more than a garnish. Its flavones and carotenoids, particularly lutein, zeaxanthin, and beta-carotene make it worth using more often to flavor soups and stews, salads, meat dishes, pasta, rice, and anything else that needs a splash of green. Italian parsley, also called flat-leaf parsley, is a common component in many Italian dishes and is now widely available. Although more commonly featured in Mexican cuisine, cilantro is a relative of parsley. Both contain immune system–boosting polyacetylenes.

- **Chili peppers.** The ingredient in cayenne or hot pepper, chili peppers contain a phytochemical called capsaicin, thought to fight cancer and possibly decrease pain. Chili peppers also contain carotenoids, including lutein, zeaxanthin, and beta-carotene, and a dose of vitamin C. Use chili peppers to spice up any dish. Although chili peppers are more familiar in the cuisines of non-Mediterranean cultures such as Mexico and India, cayenne pepper (dried ground chili pepper) is widely used in North African cuisine. Authentic or not, add zip to paella, gazpacho, fish or shrimp, and eggs with chili peppers.

- **Turmeric.** Brilliant yellow turmeric is used extensively in Indian and southeast Asian cuisine, but is also a component of many African dishes. Turmeric contains the phytochemical curcumin, a phenolic compound with powerful antioxidant effects.

The above is just a sampling of the many herbs and spices used in Mediterranean cuisine. Experiment with herbs and spices to broaden your culinary spectrum and add both intense flavor and a phytochemical boost to your favorite foods.

✆ *Are sun-dried tomatoes as nutritious as fresh tomatoes?*

Yes. Just like a raisin is as nutritious as a grape, the sun-dried tomato is full of lycopene and contains all the nutrients of a vine-ripe tomato. The only element missing is the water. The sun-dried tomato also contains the same number of calories as a fresh tomato. However, because it is smaller, it is easier to eat more sun-dried tomatoes than fresh tomatoes. Of course, the calories in vegetables are minimal and these are calories with nutritional power, so no need to limit yourself. Sun-dried tomatoes make a flavorful addition to many dishes and are even a tasty addition to homemade bread.

❦ Are frozen vegetables as nutritious as fresh vegetables?

Not always, but sometimes the frozen version of your favorite veggie is actually *more* nutritious than the fresh version. Many vegetables are flash-frozen and bagged right in the field after picking, preserving many nutrients that might otherwise be destroyed by rough handling and extreme temperatures, not to mention plain old exposure to the air during the long transport to your local supermarket and finally to your refrigerator. Some nutrients are easily oxidized and depleted during this trek.

That's not to say you shouldn't seek out fresh produce! Seek out local produce stands or, better yet, grow your own vegetables. The trip from garden to dinner plate is much shorter, and you'll be getting the best flavor and most nutritional value possible. When good fresh produce isn't available, however, you can rest assured that frozen and canned vegetables are a pretty close second when it comes to nutritional value.

❦ How much folacin is in different kinds of foods?

Many kinds of beans, vegetables, fruit, whole grains, nuts, and seeds contain folacin. All of these foods are recommended to be consumed on a daily basis in the Mediterranean Diet Pyramid, making it easy to get adequate amounts of folacin. The recommended daily allowance for the average adult is 180 to 200 micrograms. Women in childbearing years, and those who are pregnant, are recommended to get 400 micrograms of folacin per day. Some researchers feel that folacin intakes should be from 400 to 800 micrograms per day to help prevent cancer. Below is a chart of some foods and their folacin content:

Food	Folacin (micrograms)
Artichoke, *boiled (1 medium)*	155
Asparagus, *boiled (1/2 cup, or 6 spears)*	130
Avocado, raw *(1 medium)*	160
Blackberries *(frozen, unsweetened, 1 cup)*	50
Boysenberries *(frozen, unsweetened, 1 cup)*	85
Broccoli, raw *(1/2 cup chopped)*	30
Chickpeas (garbanzo beans), *boiled (1 cup)*	280
Orange juice *(8 ounces)*	110
Red kidney beans, *boiled (1 cup)*	230
Rye flour, *dark (1 cup)*	80
Sunflower seeds, *toasted (1 oz)*	65
Turnip greens, *boiled (1/2 cup, chopped)*	85

Food	*Folacin (micrograms)*
Whole wheat, wheat flour (1 cup)	55

*Note: These figures are rounded numbers. Source: Pennington, Jean. 1998. Bowes & Churches, Food Values of Portions Commonly Used, (17ed). Philadelphia: Lippincott.

✣ RECIPES

🌾 RATATOUILLE

This traditional vegetable dish from the Provençal region combines eggplant, tomatoes, peppers, and zucchini in a brilliant mosaic of colors and textures, but feel free to substitute other fresh seasonal vegetables in your own kitchen. Seasonality is the key to authenticity.

Ratatouille is often served as an accompaniment to meat or fish. We like it as a main course served with a rice (saffron-tinted yellow rice is perfect). It is so beautiful that all the other food goes unnoticed anyway!

A note about eggplant: Some people like to salt eggplant and let it sit in a colander for 30 to 60 minutes to draw out any bitterness. Very fresh young eggplant, heavy for its size without blemishes and with a tight skin that bounces back after being lightly pressed, shouldn't be bitter, but feel free to salt if you are wary of bitterness.

We tried to keep this recipe relatively low in oil. A nonstick skillet will make it much easier to keep this dish lower in fat. If veggies really start to stick, however (if you are cooking in cast iron, for example), you may need to increase the amount of olive oil somewhat.

1 medium onion, coarsely chopped
1 large red bell pepper, cut into squares
1 large green, yellow, or orange bell pepper, cut into
    squares
4 cloves garlic, chopped
6 tablespoons extra-virgin olive oil
1 medium or two small, very fresh eggplants, peeled
    and cut into 1-inch cubes
1 medium zucchini, cut into 1-inch cubes
1 small hot chili pepper, chopped, or a dash of
    cayenne pepper (optional)
2 cups peeled, chopped, and seeded ripe tomatoes
    (about 2 medium—to peel, immerse tomatoes for
    about 30 seconds in boiling water to loosen the
    skins) or one 15-ounce can tomatoes
½ teaspoon sugar
1 bay leaf
¼ cup chopped fresh basil
¼ cup pitted ripe olives, sliced or chopped

In a large skillet, sauté the onion, bell peppers, and garlic in 2 tablespoons of the olive oil until all are soft but not browned. Remove from the skillet and set aside.

Add another 2 tablespoons of the oil to the skillet and sauté the eggplant cubes until golden brown and tender (it takes about 10 minutes). Eggplant is an oil sponge so rather than continuing to add oil, keep stirring to prevent sticking. Remove the eggplant from the skillet and set aside with the onion-pepper mixture (you can combine them in a single bowl).

Add the remaining 2 tablespoons of oil and sauté the zucchini and chili pepper, if you are using it (if you are using cayenne pepper, don't add it yet), until the zucchini is tender and golden. Remove from the skillet and set aside (again, you can add them to the bowl of other vegetables).

You should have some oil remaining in the pan. If you don't, add another teaspoon, then add the tomatoes and sugar, and the cayenne pepper if you are using it. Lower the heat and simmer, stirring frequently, for about 15 minutes, or until the tomatoes are reduced to a thick jamlike consistency.

Gently add the cooked vegetables you have set aside, stirring them into the tomatoes. Warm through (about five minutes), then stir in the fresh basil and black olives. Serve over or beside rice.

Makes about 4 servings.

Nutritional information per serving (roughly): 355 calories, 20 grams total fat (3 grams saturated fat, 13 grams monounsaturated fat) (Note: Reduce the calories and fat by using a nonstick skillet to prepare this recipe.)

✒ GREEK SALAD

A traditional Greek salad made with fresh produce and kalamata (as opposed to the so-called Spanish) olives is a culinary experience not to be missed. Served on a platter, it is an impressive addition to the dinner table. We've chosen to leave out the traditional anchovies, but feel free to add a few anchovy fillets along with the olives if you fancy them.

This salad is most transcendent if you purchase the best and freshest ingredients. Savor every bite!

> *2 cups bite-sized pieces romaine lettuce*
> *2 medium tomatoes, cut into wedges*
> *½ cup thinly sliced red onions*
> *½ cup thinly sliced cucumbers (cut them into half-circles if they are too large to be bite-sized)*
> *½ cup thinly sliced green bell peppers*

½ cup thinly sliced red bell peppers
1 tablespoon minced fresh Italian (flat-leaf) parsley
½ cup crumbled good-quality feta cheese
10 pitted kalamata or other good-quality Greek olives

Dressing:

¼ cup extra-virgin olive oil
1 tablespoon fresh lemon juice
1 small clove garlic, minced
½ teaspoon minced fresh oregano (or ¼ teaspoon dried oregano, crushed)

Spread the romaine lettuce on a roomy platter. Arrange the tomato wedges over the lettuce. In a bowl, combine the onions, cucumbers, peppers, Italian parsley, and half the feta cheese, then spread over the lettuce and tomatoes. Top with the olives and remaining feta cheese.

To make the dressing, whisk together the oil, lemon juice, garlic, and oregano, then drizzle over the salad. Toss just before serving.

Makes about 4 servings.

Nutritional information per serving (roughly): 295 calories, 25 grams total fat (7 grams saturated fat, 14 grams monounsaturated fat) (Note: Reduce the fat and calories in the above recipe by using a reduced-fat or low-fat feta cheese and decreasing the amount of olives and olive oil.)

🌾 STUFFED ARTICHOKES

This dish can be an entrée (one artichoke per person) or a side dish to accompany a pasta, rice, bean, or fish dish (one artichoke for two to share). This recipe may sound complicated, but once you are familiar with preparing artichokes, it really is easy. It also looks terribly impressive and is sure to elicit "oohs" and "ahhs" from appreciative diners.

This dish hails from Italy and is prepared in the fall, when artichokes are in season. Look for artichokes that are a bright green with firm, plump leaves.

> 2 cups fresh (not dry) whole-grain bread crumbs
> 1 cup grated Parmesan, Romano, or Pecorino cheese
> 1 medium onion, finely chopped
> 3 cloves garlic, minced
> 2 tablespoons minced fresh Italian (flat-leaf) parsley
> 4 large artichokes
> Fresh lemon juice
> ½ cup extra-virgin olive oil
> 4 lemon wedges

In a large bowl, combine the bread crumbs, grated cheese, onion, garlic, and parsley. Set aside.

Rinse the artichokes and drain well. Prepare the artichokes by cutting off the top ½ inch with a very sharp knife. Brush immediately with a little fresh lemon juice. Cut off the stems so that the artichokes will sit upright in the pan and brush the bottoms with lemon juice. Snip off the sharp tips of the leaves with scissors and remove any very tough outer leaves. Brush all cut surfaces with lemon juice.

Spread the artichoke leaves and, using a spoon or your fingers, stuff the bread-crumb mixture among as many leaves as you can, dividing the mixture among the four artichokes.

Carefully place the artichokes in a saucepan or Dutch oven. Drizzle the olive oil evenly over the four artichokes. Boil some water in a teakettle or saucepan and add enough hot water to cover the bottom third of the artichokes, pouring carefully to avoid getting water on the filling (some filling is bound to spill out throughout the entire process, but do your best). Heat the artichokes until the water boils again, then lower the heat and simmer about 30 to 40 minutes or until the artichokes are tender.

Remove the artichokes carefully to a platter and serve with lemon wedges.

Makes 4 servings.

Nutritional information per serving: 1,055 calories, 50 grams total fat (16 grams saturated fat, 28 grams monounsaturated fat)

🌿 GAZPACHO

This Spanish favorite is hard for some to comprehend. Cold soup? And why not? Gazpacho is loaded with nutritious, fresh vegetables and has a sparkling fresh taste with just a hint of spice—the perfect remedy for a torrid summer day, especially if you are feeling too lazy even to chew.

Traditional gazpacho often includes bread ground into the soup, but we prefer a more intense vegetable flavor and like to make this soup *sans* bread.

3 cups peeled, chopped ripe tomatoes (about 3 medium—to peel, immerse tomatoes for about 30 seconds in boiling water to loosen the skins)
1 clove garlic, minced
½ cup chopped red onion
½ cup chopped bell pepper (any color)
½ cup peeled, chopped cucumber
½ cup extra-virgin olive oil
1 tablespoon good-quality wine vinegar

½ cup water with enough ice cubes added to make
   1 cup
¼ teaspoon ground cumin
Dash of cayenne pepper

In the bowl of a food processor fitted with the metal blade or blender container, combine all the ingredients and process until smooth. Serve from a pitcher on the veranda, or take it to the beach!

Makes about 4 servings.

Nutritional information per serving (roughly): 319 calories, 30 grams total fat (4 grams saturated fat, 20 grams monounsaturated fat) (Note: For a low-fat variation, use only ½ cup of grated cheese and 4 tablespoons of olive oil.)

5: *The Fruits of Good Health*

Who can resist a perfectly ripe piece of fruit? Tender, blushing peaches; rosy slices of watermelon; mahogany plums dripping with garnet-colored juice; crisp, crunchy apples; luscious, sunny oranges; sweet, mellow bananas; succulent berries in a rainbow of hues. Few things are more pleasurable than eating really good fruit. So why don't we eat more, and why do we so often fall short of the recommended absolute minimum of two servings of fruit per day? Why do Americans seem to prefer a box of store-bought cookies or cake from a mix for dessert?

In the traditional Mediterranean diet, fruit is a meal's crowning glory, the ultimate finish to a delicious dinner. The Mediterranean climate is perfect for growing a wide variety of fruits, and whatever is freshest, juiciest, most lovely, and in season provides the final flourish to meals already rich in color, texture, flavor, vitamins, minerals, fiber, phytonutrients, and good old-fashioned pleasure.

Fruits are full of great nutrition. Most fruits are high in that ever-helpful and healthful antioxidant vitamin C (for more on the antioxidant powers of vitamin C, see the previous chapter). All fruits are full of essential vitamins and minerals, as well as fiber (more on fiber in Chapter Six). Many contain high doses of carotenoids and other phytochemicals such as caffeic acid and coumarins, which help the body to rid itself of carcinogens; ferulic acid, which may help to shuttle potentially carcinogenic nitrates out of the body; cryptoxanthin, a carotenoid associated with decreased cervical cancer risk; and flavonoids.

Additionally, many studies have linked high fruit consumption (in conjunction with high vegetable consumption or on its own) with lower rates of certain cancers. A study published in the *American Journal of Clinical Nutrition* examined the specific effect of fruit consumption on cancer, and found "strong protective effects . . . for cancers of the upper digestive and respiratory tracts," as well as a lesser effect "on cancers of the oral cavity, pharynx, esophagus, and larynx." The study also found that the farther a tumor was from the digestive tract, the weaker the protective effect of fruit. Nonetheless, the study also found "significant protective effects of fruit . . . for cancers of the liver, pancreas, prostate, and urinary tract."

Yet, despite fruit's demonstrated healthfulness and great taste, in America, eating desserts higher in both refined sugar and fat than a simple piece of fruit seems to be the norm. A fancy pastry, a chocolate sundae, or candy bar are weekly, even daily treats for many. Such high-sugar, high-fat fare is only an occasional treat in the traditional Mediterranean diet, never a daily or even a weekly indulgence.

While people in some parts of the Mediterranean enjoy a small bite of something sweet during the late afternoon, rich desserts never follow a meal, and portions are relatively tiny. Fruit appropriately follows a heavily plant-based meal, offering both the fulfillment of that desire for something sweet, fiber to provide a feeling of satiety, and one last dose of nutrients and phytochemicals to send the diner on his or her way.

While a ripe, juicy piece of raw fruit is the ultimate treat, fruit can also be delicious cooked, stewed, or added to recipes. Check out the recipe section of this chapter for some Mediterranean-inspired ideas.

Many of the fruits listed below have been enjoyed for centuries in the Mediterranean. A few are native to North America, or are more often consumed here than elsewhere. While we will mention the availability of each of the following fruits in the Mediterranean, the important point we would like to make is that any high-quality, ripe, juicy, fresh fruit available to you is appropriate for your diet, and finishing your meals with any fruit is to eat in the true Mediterranean spirit.

℅ APPLES

Apples are a part of the cuisines of many countries, and have existed in the Mediterranean as early as the third century B.C., when Cato, a Roman writer, mentioned seven different varieties of apples. The Roman Pliny, writing in the first century A.D., names thirty-six varieties of apples in his writings. Caesar's invading Roman legions are credited with introducing apples to Britain, and the first American settlers brought apple seeds to the New World.

One medium apple has about 80 calories and supplies 5 grams of fiber, more than a serving of oatmeal and about one fourth the daily fiber recommended by the American Dietetic Association. Most of the fiber in apples is soluble fiber, a substance demonstrated to lower cholesterol levels. But the benefits don't stop there. A daily apple may indeed keep the doctor away, especially if that daily apple remains unpeeled.

Recent research out of Cornell University has uncovered a host of phytochemicals in apple skins, including the flavonoids known as quercetin glycoside, phloretin glycoside, chlorogenic acid, and epicatechin, most heavily concentrated in the skin. Apples have been shown to exhibit higher antioxidant activity than oranges, grapefruits, carrots, spinach, onions, and green peppers, according to the Cornell study. (Wash and rinse apples well with dish soap and water if they aren't organically grown.)

Yet, Americans only eat, on average, an apple every three days. Apples are one of the hardier fruits that keep well, ship well, and compared to many fruits, are amazingly long-lived. This durability adds to apples' convenience. You can buy them in bulk and eat them, as long as they are stored in a cool, dry place, for months. Some apples can keep for six months or more (such as the popular Red Delicious) under the right conditions. What food could be more convenient than an apple?

Look for apples with firm flesh and without bruises, soft spots, depressions, cuts and nicks, or little holes. If the inside flesh is showing and has been exposed to the air, vitamins and minerals may have been destroyed. Apples grown locally or regionally are great if you can get them. Big or small, apples can be surprisingly sweet and juicy. Color varies among apple varieties. Red Delicious, for example, are a bright or deep red, while Gala apples are yellow overlaid with a rosier red.

Avoid apples with a brilliant shine. Lots of shine probably means lots of wax, which traps pesticides. If you can find only waxed apples, peel them before eating. Whether you peel or not, wash all apples with soap and a scrub brush. Cut out any bruises or nicks. Apples last longer in the refrigerator and ripen faster at room temperature (as is the case with many fruits).

Some of the more widely available apple types, all

great for eating out of hand, are Braeburn, Empire, Fuji, Gala, Golden Delicious, Granny Smith (also perfect for pies), Jonagold, Jonathan, McIntosh, Red Delicious, Rome Beauty (also ideal for baking), and Winesap. Many other types exist too. Check your local market, produce stand, or grocery store. Apples are widely available all year round in the United States, and the many types, flavors, colors, and uses make them irresistible. Shouldn't you be eating more?

℅ APRICOTS

Apricots are familiar to denizens of the Mediterranean, particularly in Turkey. Americans like their apricots fresh, canned, and dried, and each form has its gastronomical and nutritional benefits. The bright orange-yellow color is a dead giveaway that these velvety little fruits are potent sources of beta-carotene in any form. Dried apricots are a concentrated source of energy and fiber, as well as many other essential vitamins and minerals. Fresh apricots are richer in vitamin C, and when eaten at the peak of ripeness and slightly warmed by the sun, are an utter delight.

The problem with fresh apricots is that they are incredibly delicate and don't last long. The apricot season in the United States is approximately May through July, but if apricots aren't grown near you, you may have trouble finding good fresh ones. Ripe apricots are soft and have a lovely apricot aroma. If apricots are greenish when picked, they will probably spoil before they ripen, but you can attempt to ripen them by storing them at room temperature in a brown paper bag. Dried apricots and cooked or canned apricots are other delicious and nutritious alternatives.

❦ BANANAS

Although you may not think of bananas as being a typical Mediterranean fruit, bananas are a part of the cuisines of Africa and Spain. Descriptions of bananas can be found in Greek texts from the time of Alexander the Great. Spanish missionaries introduced bananas to many parts of the world, and these cousins of the lily (which, incidentally, grow on very tall plants, not trees) exist in many forms and types throughout the world.

Conveniently wrapped in their own package, bananas are known to be good sources of potassium, that mineral needed for our heart to beat normally. When potassium levels fall dangerously low, which can happen during fasting or with severe diarrhea or vomiting, sudden death can occur. Potassium is also involved in maintaining our body's fluid balance and keeping our cells healthy. (Oranges, dates, and figs are actually richer sources of potassium than bananas.)

Bananas are delicious when the tips are still green, when the flavor is tangier, and at every stage until the skins are quite dark. The riper the banana, the sweeter it tastes. Cooked bananas are even sweeter, and grilled bananas are a delicious dessert, or even a side dish with a main course. Firmer, less ripe bananas are best for grilling or frying, while very ripe bananas mashed to a pulp are a superb addition to baked goods, and can even take the place of some of the fat.

❦ BERRIES

What a glorious category of fruit! Berries are colorful, fun to eat, juicy, delicious, even fun to pick. They are perfect for cooking or eating raw. Freeze them for an icy treat, bake them into bread, or pop them one after another for a snack. Berries are delicate and they don't last long, so buy them, rinse them, and eat them immediately—and often.

Berries are beloved in the Mediterranean. Fragrant wild strawberries are a much-anticipated component of produce markets in Italy, and although the strawberries cultivated in the United States are somewhat different, the spirit remains the same. Blueberries, cultivated in North America, make a lovely Mediterranean-type dessert and are reminiscent of their cousins, the lingonberries, the blueberry's European (and Mediterranean) equivalent. Plump, juicy blackberries, tangy raspberries, tart, globe-shaped gooseberries, and the all-American cranberry are other delicious choices. (Cranberries are too tart to eat raw for most people, but they are wonderful cooked into recipes.)

The vibrant colors of berries are a giveaway that these juicy fruits, perfect for snacking, are loaded with cancer-fighting phytochemicals. Flavonoids make blackberries purple-black, blueberries deep blue, and strawberries and raspberries rosy red. Berries are also full of vitamin C, fiber, and folate, all cancer fighters, too. In fact, in the fight against cancer, few foods are more powerful than berries.

Unlike some fruits, berries will last only a day or two in your refrigerator, and a little mold on one berry can transform the whole bowlful into a moldy mess overnight. Even berries untouched by the mold can take on an unpleasant taste. The best choice is to pick your own berries or buy them from a local produce stand or farmer's market. Alternatively, berries from the supermarket can be stored layered between paper towels, and lightly rinsed just before serving. Blueberries last slightly longer than other types, such as strawberries, blackberries, and raspberries. Firmer and best used in cooking, cranberries are the exception. They keep well in the refrigerator and will keep for months in the freezer. When you can't find them fresh, frozen berries are similarly high in nutrients.

❦ CHERRIES

Although the cherry tree's unfortunate fate at the hands of little Georgie Washington is the stuff of American legend, cherries have been around for centuries and were probably first domesticated over two-thousand years ago in southern Turkey or Greece. The Romans loved them and they have been planted and consumed all over Europe for centuries.

The cherry varieties most available in the United States are sweet cherries—the popular, mahogany-skinned Bing cherry, the yellow-pink Rainier cherry, the dark red Lambert cherry, and the sweet Vans cherry—and sour cherries, most often used in pie fillings and other cooked desserts. Gaining in popularity are tart-sweet dried cherries.

Cherries are in season in midsummer and arrive at the market fully ripe. They are best handled gently, washed right before eating (when feasible—if not, wash and pat dry, then store in the refrigerator), and eaten as soon as possible. Choose plump, glossy berries with deep color and strong, intact stems. If you don't plan to eat your cherries right away, store them in the refrigerator, as you would berries, unrinsed between layers of paper towels, then wrap in plastic or store in an airtight container. Rinse just before serving.

Cherries are rich in quercetin and kaempferol (flavinols), plus other powerful antioxidants. Tart cherries may also have anti-inflammatory properties, making them possible allies in the fight against arthritis pain (the Cherry Marketing Institute suggests eating twenty tart cherries per day to reduce inflammatory pain).

❦ CITRUS FRUIT

Citrus fruit is plentiful in America, grown in abundance in Florida, Arizona, and California. It travels well, keeps well, and is plentiful all year in every state, making it a convenient (and self-packaged) food. Citrus trees are also familiar fixtures in the Mediterranean, as the climate is just right. Therefore, including lots of fresh oranges, grapefruits, tangerines, lemons, and limes in your diet is quintessentially Mediterranean. And don't forget the more unusual citrus choices, for variety: kumquats, tangelos, and tangors.

The orange juice industry has made it known that orange juice contains the folic acid so important for women of childbearing age. Deficiencies of folic acid have been linked to fetal abnormalities, and the United States Food and Drug Administration has stated that women of childbearing age can dramatically reduce the risk of having a child with neural tube defects such as spina bifida and anencephaly by consuming enough fruits and vegetables to assure adequate folic acid intake. Although some legumes and vegetables are even richer sources of folic acid, the orange still ranks as a good source.

Citrus fruits' real claim to fame is its high concentration of the antioxidant vitamin C. Although vitamin C is present in most fruits, one medium orange supplies the entire recommended daily allowance (currently 60 milligrams, although recent studies have suggested that 100 to 200 milligrams daily best saturates cells with vitamin C). Many studies have linked vitamin C consumption with reduced cancer risk. In addition to vitamin C's antioxidant properties (discussed in detail in the previous chapter), vitamin C gives the immune system a boost and aids the body in the absorption of iron, particularly that from plant-based sources, which aren't as readily absorbed by the body as the iron in animal meats. If you down a glass of orange juice with your iron-fortified cereal (for an extra C-boost, throw in a few strawberries, too), your body will absorb more iron than it would without the extra vitamin C (for more on iron, see Chapter Seven).

Vitamin C is also important for maintaining the body's collagen supply. Collagen is necessary for healing wounds, strengthening blood vessels, and maintaining bones and teeth. Collagen has also been linked to a decreased risk of cancer metastasizing (spreading through the body).

Too much vitamin C (in daily megadoses of over 1,000 milligrams) could lead to kidney stone formation in certain people, and even higher doses have been shown to cause abdominal cramping, diarrhea, and nausea. Such megadoses would be virtually impossible to achieve from food, and are only a problem when people take vitamin C supplements, so we recommend getting your vitamin C from food sources—and what better food source than citrus fruits?

In addition to vitamin C, citrus fruit has other star qualities. Red grapefruit has been the subject of recent cancer research because of its high level of lycopene, the phytochemical that has been linked to lower rates of prostate and possibly breast and colon cancer. Red grapefruit is sweeter than yellow grapefruit, just one more reason to enjoy it. Even those who don't normally appreciate grapefruit's puckering tang might enjoy the sweeter red variety.

Don't worry about the color of the rind when choosing your citrus. Most commercially produced citrus is waxed and much of it is dyed. The citrus rind and citrus oil are also potent sources of the phytochemical limonene, a monoterpene often used in household products like detergent and furniture polish (which you should not, of course, eat!). Limonene has exhibited extremely strong anticancer effects, even causing complete regression of mammary tumors in laboratory rats. Try slicing organic citrus rind and candying it for a unique treat, made even more special when dipped in chocolate (for special occasions only—despite the orange rind, this is basically candy). Many cookbooks contain recipes for candied lemon, orange, and grapefruit peels.

Store citrus fruits in the refrigerator to keep them fresh the longest. Citrus can also be stored in a cool, dry place but will need to be eaten more quickly. Make sure the citrus can breathe. Airtight bags or containers tend to encourage molding. If allowed to come to room temperature, citrus fruits will be juicier and more fragrant.

✺ GRAPES

Whether or not you are a fan of wine, you very well may be a fan of the noble grape. Whether green, red, or blue-black, grapes are fun to eat, deliciously juicy, and as sweet a fruit as anyone could wish for. Grapes are one of the oldest cultivated fruits known to man, and hieroglyphic evidence exists that the people of ancient Egypt were growing grapes and making wine.

Some grapes are native to North America, but the

Mediterranean region was the first to cultivate grapes, transforming them from small, sour fruits to the juicy globes of sweetness we know and love today. European grapes brought to North America from Europe sparked the consumption of fresh grapes, the making of raisins, and the California wine culture.

Even today, Italy leads the world in the production of table grapes. (Chile is second and California is third.) However, in the United States, 97 percent of the table grapes available come from California. Other states producing grapes include Arizona, Michigan, and New York. The most popular eating grape in this country is Thompson seedless, a delicious variety of green grape. Because it is seedless, Thompson grapes (and other seedless varieties) are exceptionally convenient snack foods.

Grapes are available all year, adding to their convenience. They are harvested ripe, so choose any grapes that look plump and fresh, are firmly attached to their stems, and have a healthy bloom (the white powdery cast to fresh grapes). Green grapes should have a golden cast, and red and blue-black grapes should have a deep, even color. Grapes brought to room temperature before serving are the most flavorful. Rinse just before serving.

Grapes (especially the red varieties) are rich sources of flavonoids, the substances in wine suspected to offer so many health benefits (see page 147 for more on wine). Grapes also contain caffeic, ferulic, and ellagic acids, phenolic acids with strong antioxidant properties that give both grapes and wine their color and flavor as well as the characteristic tartness. Grapes additionally contain the phytoestrogen resveratrol, a phenolic fungicide that may support a healthy heart. (Peanuts also contain resveratrol.)

A small bunch of fresh grapes makes a satisfying conclusion to any meal. Raisins are also great for snacking, in breads, and in recipes where fruit is cooked.

✥ MELONS

A highly perfumed melon evokes ancient times in exotic lands. Native to Africa and first cultivated there, the first recorded watermelon harvesting was nearly five-thousand years ago in Egypt, according to the National Watermelon Promotion Board. Pharaohs stocked watermelons in their tombs, and legend has it that the Roman governor Demosthenes, after ducking half a watermelon that was thrown at him during a political debate, set the watermelon on his head and thanked the thrower for the helmet to wear while fighting Philip of Macedonia.

Watermelons are thought to have grown along the banks of the Nile even before 2000 B.C., and cantaloupe seeds brought from Armenia as a gift to the Pope were first planted in Cantalupo, Italy—hence, their contemporary name. Melons of all types spread all over the Mediterranean region centuries ago and have been a part of the Mediterranean diet ever since. Whether for dessert or wrapped in slices of prosciutto as an antipasto, melons are a Mediterranean favorite. While the melons grown in the Mediterranean aren't widely available in this country (such as the dark green Spanish melon), other melons, such as juicy cantaloupe and honeydew melons, are available during much of the year, although they are in season in late summer through fall. Once only available during the summer when they are in season, watermelons are now also available all year, depending on where you live.

To pick a perfect honeydew or cantaloupe, look for a fruit with a pleasing melony scent at the smooth end. It should yield slightly to pressure at the stem end and be heavy for its size without cracks or spots. Cantaloupe should have a golden netting over light yellow. Honeydew melons should be creamy white or light yellow in color with a slightly oily film on the outer rind. Melons that stand for a couple of days at room temperature will be juicier and more aromatic.

Watermelons should also seem heavy for their size and their bottom side should be pale yellow, signifying that the watermelon ripened on the ground. Folklore suggests balancing a broom straw on top of a watermelon to determine ripeness. If the straw rotates slowly, the melon is ripe.

Melons are heavy on nutrition. They contain many vitamins and minerals, as well as fiber. The watermelon's red color is the result of the powerful antioxidant carotenoid lycopene, that cancer fighter also present in tomatoes and red grapefruit thought to reduce prostate cancer risk and possibly breast cancer risk. Cantaloupe is high in vitamin C and beta-carotene (obvious from its orange color). Honeydew melons are also good sources of vitamin C.

Although melons do not cook well, raw melons make a lovely dessert or even as part of the main meal, served in slices, cubes, or balls alongside meat or grain-based dishes. For a truly Mediterranean appetizer, serve slender cantaloupe and honeydew slices wrapped in strips of prosciutto (an admittedly pricey dry-cured Italian ham), pancetta (an unsmoked salt-cured Italian bacon), or if you are looking for more accessible ingredients, Canadian bacon or thinly sliced ham. All versions are tasty.

℘ PEACHES AND NECTARINES

Peaches and nectarines (a smooth-skinned type of peach) are spectacular summer fruits when you are lucky enough to get good ones. In the Mediterranean, where peaches are abundant in the summer, the quality is high. In the United States, peaches and nectarines bought out of season are frequently disappointing, even inedible. Nothing compares to the perfect, juicy, fragrant peach or nectarine, however. These fruits don't need any adornment.

However, peaches stuffed with chopped nuts and the crumbs of almond cookies are a popular Italian dish (see the recipe section later in the chapter), and fresh peaches or nectarines poached in a little wine are a not-so-sinful pleasure, considering the high nutritional content of these fruits: rich in vitamin C, beta-carotene, and other carotenoids (again, the color is the clue), peaches and nectarines are a nutritious way to wind up a great meal. Cooking brings out even more of the flavor in even the ripest peach, so consider cooking peaches whenever the mood strikes you. In addition to poaching, peaches are delicious grilled, baked, or even lightly sautéed in a fruity olive or nut oil. Peaches are closely related to almonds, so any combination of these two "fruits" is exceptionally pleasing.

Peaches and nectarines don't keep well, but will keep longer, once ripe, in the refrigerator. Both are best purchased tree-ripened. Skin color is irrelevant to ripeness but the peach should yield slightly to light pressure and have a fruity aroma. To ripen an unripe peach or nectarine, place one to three fruits in a paper bag for two or three days. Peaches and nectarines are in season (increasing your chances of getting good ones) in July and August. When you can't find good fresh peaches or nectarines, canned and frozen peaches are an acceptable alternative, retaining most of their nutritional value (they lose some vitamin C but the carotenoid content remains the same).

❧ PEARS

Known throughout the Mediterranean for centuries, pears are second only to apples as the favored baked fruit.

Baked pears are far less common in this country, although we aren't sure why. A fresh baked pear is a mouth-watering, sweet, buttery treat, and easy to prepare (see the recipe on page 152). Ripe pears are tasty, too—juicy, sweet, fragrant, and tender.

Most pears purchased from the supermarket aren't yet ready for eating, however. Pears are far more edible when they ripen off the tree, so green pears are picked and shipped (convenient, since the unripe pears are harder and sturdier, so they travel better). Unripe pears are exceptionally long-lived, and rival apples when it comes to long-term storage potential. Chill them and they'll last and last (the harder varieties like Bosc and Comice can keep for up to 7 months). A week or so before you are ready to eat them, bring them to room temperature and ripen in a brown paper bag.

When purchasing pears, look for firm fruit without cuts, bruises, or blemishes. Superficial nicks are fine if you plan to eat the pears that week. Bruises and soft spots should be avoided. Pears need to sit for a few days to soften sufficiently for eating once you bring them home. A ripe pear yields slightly to pressure on the stem end. A ripe pear spoils quickly. Keep it in the refrigerator for a couple of days at most.

Pears are generally available all year in the United States, but their peak season is August through October. Sample the different pear varieties in most supermarkets: Anjou, Bartlett, and Bosc are among the most widely available, but you'll often see other types. Asian pears are crisper and are best in the fall.

Pears may not sport the orange color that distinguishes carotenoid-heavy fruit, but they have plenty of other nutritional properties to recommend them. Pears are full of vitamin C and fresh raw pears are particularly high in fiber. They also contain many other vitamins and minerals. Dried pears are great for snacking and are a more concentrated source of nutrients.

✿ PLUMS

Plums are no strangers to the traditional Mediterranean diet. Spiced plums cooked with sugar, cinnamon, and cloves is a French specialty, served chilled. Many types of plums are available in the United States, including the juicy Japanese plums perfect for snacking and the drier European plums best suited for cooking. Plums are available from May through October.

Plums range in color from yellow to blue-black, with every shade of red, purple, and blue in between. Plums are best when tree-ripened, but because plums soften (without developing additional sweetness) after picking, ripe and unripe plums can both feel soft and ripe in the store. If your market allows it, you will be better off taste-testing the store's plums before buying. Plums are a nutritious and complexly flavored dessert.

Let us not forget plums in their dried form! Super-nutritious prunes have a reputation for promoting regularity, but they do far more than provide fiber for our bodies. Prunes are a concentrated source of many vitamins and minerals, and have high levels of caffeic and ferulic acid, phenolic acids demonstrated to have potent anticancer effects in animal studies.

✿ THE GREAT WINE CONTROVERSY

On November 17, 1991, a segment aired on the popular television show *60 Minutes* that changed the world—or at least, the world as wine fanciers and wine producers know it. The show examined the diets, lifestyles, and health of people living in southwestern France, where saturated fat intake (primarily from butter, cream, and cheese) was high. The surprising finding was the low heart attack rate among the French—one of the lowest in the world! This discovery flew in the face of everything the American public had been told about how to lower the risk of coronary heart disease. What were the French doing to keep their heart attack rates so low? The study concluded that they were drinking wine.

Hallelujah, the world responded! We can eat whatever we want, follow it with a glass of wine, and everyone will be fine! Within a few weeks of the airing of the notorious *60 Minutes* episode, red wine sales rose 40 percent in the United States.

Of course, like any purported panacea, the picture is far more complicated than it seems at first glance. While wine does appear to have many benefits, from a high flavonoid content to antibacterial effects, the French study subjects didn't overindulge. Red wine consumption in France is, on average, daily but moderate—about 8 ounces per day for men, half that amount at most for women.

One study out of Denmark suggests that wine drinkers tend to have better eating habits. Wine drinkers, according to the study, tended to eat more fruits and vegetables, fish, salads, and olive oil, making the health benefits of wine a little less clear. Research in the United States additionally suggests that wine drinkers are, in general, more moderate drinkers who smoke less and are better educated.

Alcohol consumption of any kind has been linked to increased risk of breast cancer in women, so women may think twice about a daily glass of wine. One study suggests that two to five drinks a day can increase a woman's risk of developing breast cancer by 40 percent. While the recommended single 4-ounce daily serving of wine (red or white) may be small enough to make little difference in cancer risk, those otherwise at risk for breast cancer needn't feel compelled to drink any.

Anyone at risk for alcohol-related problems should also forego wine in favor of more fruits and vegetables. Alcohol intake has been associated with an increased risk of accidents and all causes of death, and alcohol is certainly not a necessary component in any healthy diet. While many researchers suspect flavonoids are the key to the protection wine may offer against heart disease, plenty of other fruits and vegetables have more flavonoids than a glass of wine (see chart on page 150).

For those who already enjoy wine in moderation, however, the research investigating the link between wine consumption and health is intriguing. Research has shown a U-shaped curve linking alcohol consumption with longevity. People who drink alcohol in moderation seem to enjoy a longer life than people who don't drink at all or people who drink heavily. "Moderation" generally refers to two or fewer 8-ounce glasses of wine per day for men, and less than one 8-ounce glass of wine for women.

Although some research suggests a longer life for moderate alcohol drinkers, alcohol consumption certainly has its risks, and other studies dispute the claim that moderate drinkers live any longer than nondrinkers.

The link between wine consumption and a reduced risk of heart disease is even more compelling. Many studies have associated moderate alcohol intake with improved cardiovascular health, especially a reduced risk of suffering a heart attack, and much research has been conducted in an attempt to determine what particular aspects of alcohol and/or wine consumption are responsible for this protective effect. One theory is that

alcohol has a protective tendency to raise HDL ("good")
cholesterol and lower LDL ("bad") cholesterol; another
centers on alcohol's tendency to inhibit blood clotting.
Other researchers are investigating wine's particular
antioxidant phytochemicals, specifically phenolic compounds like flavonoids and the phenolic fungicide
resveratrol.

Keep in mind, however, that most plant foods contain
phenolic compounds, many in concentrations higher than
in wine. Grapes and peanuts are also good sources of
resveratrol, and flavonoids are present in many plant
foods, especially red grapes, green leafy vegetables, and
fruity vegetables like tomatoes. If these antioxidant compounds are the "magic ingredient" in wine, then consumption of grapes and other foods with high levels of
phenolic compounds should offer similar protection. The
following chart demonstrates the relative flavonoid content of various fruits and vegetables.

Flavonoid Content	Beverage	Fruit	Vegetable
Low flavonoid content (<10mg/kg or mg/L)	Coffee Orange Juice White Wine	Peaches	Cabbage Carrots Mush- rooms Peas Spinach
Moderate flavonoid content (10-50 mg/kg or mg/L)	Red Wine Tea Tomato Juice	Apples Grapes Strawberries	Broad beans Lettuce Red peppers Tomatoes

High flavonoid content (>50mg/kg or mg/L)	None	Cranberries	Broccoli Celery Endive French beans Kale Onions

Table adapted from "Alternative approaches to lowering cholesterol" published in Patient Care, Nov. 15, 1995, v29, n18, p110(21).

The problem with wine consumption involves the American tendency to do everything in a big way, and also to choose only those aspects of a healthy program for eating or living that are most desirable. The traditional Mediterranean diet is most effective and beneficial for health if followed completely—not just red wine, olive oil, and extra bread, but all of these as part of a low-fat, plant-based diet combined with a high level of physical activity. If you enjoy wine, maximize its health benefits by consuming it in the Mediterranean way:

- Only with meals, never recreationally
- Only in small amounts—8 ounces daily for men, 4 ounces daily for women, at most
- As one part of an overall low-fat, plant-based diet and active lifestyle

Don't forget that while small amounts of daily alcohol have indeed been associated with lower risk of heart disease and other chronic health problems, as well as lower rate of death from all causes and greater longevity, consumption of larger amounts of alcohol have been linked to a higher risk of accidents, including car accidents, heart disease, certain cancers, stroke, birth defects, and an increase in death rate from all causes, not to mention alcohol dependence and a tendency toward obesity. So, to sum up, drink if you like to, but if you can't do so in moderation, abstain. *The health risks from overconsumption of alcohol far outweigh any possible lack of benefits from abstinence.*

ℬ RECIPES

✐ BAKED APPLES AND PEARS

Baked apples have a reputation for being a homey, almost old-fashioned American dessert, but why don't we ever bake pears? Both fruits are superb for baking, which brings out their flavor and transforms them into tender, melt-in-your-mouth pleasures. Baked fruit will also perfume your house as it cooks, like fruit pie with all the flavor but without the high-fat crust!

For this recipe, if you scrub the fruit well, leave the peels on. The recipe will also work with peeled fruit. You can alter this recipe to suit the taste of those you are serving—all apples, all pears, double of each, whatever seems appropriate. If you use more apples, adjust the nut and raisin amounts accordingly.

You can also use less sugar, or even none at all. If you choose to go without, you needn't alter the recipe in any way save to simply omit the sugar. Sugar brings out the taste of the baked fruit, but it isn't necessary.

This is an excellent cold-weather or winter holiday dessert.

½ cup brown sugar
¼ cup chopped walnuts, almonds, or a combination

¼ cup raisins or dried currants
4 medium to large apples
4 medium pears, still firm
1 to 2 tablespoons fresh lemon juice
2 cups red wine, apple cider, or apple juice
½ teaspoon ground cinnamon
¼ teaspoon ground nutmeg
Rind from 1 small well-washed, organically grown
    orange or lemon, cut in strips

Preheat the oven to 300 degrees.

In a small bowl, combine ¼ cup of the brown sugar, the nuts, and raisins. Set aside.

Core the apples from the top, leaving about a ½-inch of apple at the base. Don't core the pears, but slice off the very bottoms so they stand up straight. Leave their stems intact. Brush any peeled or cut fruit surfaces with lemon juice, then set the fruits upright in a 1- to 1½-quart baking pan or casserole. Stuff the apples with the nut mixture.

In a saucepan, combine the wine, cider, or juice; cinnamon; nutmeg; the remaining brown sugar; and the citrus rind. Heat to boiling, then pour carefully over the fruit. Cover the pan with a lid or aluminum foil, then bake for 30 to 45 minutes, until the fruits are soft when pierced with a fork. Baste occasionally with the wine sauce during baking.

Serve each piece of fruit in a shallow bowl or small dish with the wine sauce spooned over the top.

Makes 8 servings, or 4 for die-hard fruit lovers.

Nutritional information per serving (roughly): 345 calories, 5 grams total fat (.5 gram saturated fat, 1 gram monounsaturated fat)

✒ MACEDONIA SALAD
(A "SPIRITED" FRUIT SALAD)

One of the most beloved ways to eat fruit in the Mediterranean, besides fresh, raw, and out of hand, is to macerate it in a little wine or other alcohol. Alcohol isn't always the norm, however. Soaking fruit in a little sugar syrup or citrus juice is also a Mediterranean tradition, so choose whichever suits your taste.

Feel free to substitute equivalent amounts of your favorite fruit for any of the fruits listed below.

> *1 lemon, brought to room temperature*
> *1 cup cubed peaches or nectarines*
> *1 cup strawberries, halved, or other berries*
> *1 cup seedless grapes (green, red, or a combination)*
> *1 cup melon cubes or balls (cantaloupe, honeydew, or watermelon)*
> *¼ cup sugar (optional, but it brings out the juice)*
> *½ cup red wine or 2 tablespoons liqueur (Grand Marnier, kirsch, or amaretto are all good choices) or ½ cup orange juice*

Roll the lemon gently on the counter, then cut into quarters. Set aside.

Combine the remaining fruit gently in a large bowl and immediately squeeze each lemon quarter over the fruit, stirring gently to keep the fruit from breaking or getting mashed.

Sprinkle with the sugar then drizzle with the wine, liqueur, or orange juice. Toss gently.

Allow to sit at room temperature for 10 to 15 minutes (not more than 1 hour), then serve.

Makes about 6 servings, depending on appetites.

Nutritional information per serving (roughly): 80 calories, 0.4 gram total fat (0 grams saturated fat, 0 grams monounsaturated fat)

✒ STUFFED PEACHES

This luxurious dish is impressive and easy to prepare, not to mention delicious. Choose very fresh, large, juicy peaches for this recipe. If you really want to make it and can't find good peaches, canned peaches will work, but because they are softer, they require more delicate handling. Buy canned peaches packed in juice, not sugar syrup.

Peaches and almonds are closely related, so they make a natural pairing here. Both are also grown extensively in Italy, where baked peaches are a perennial favorite.

4 large whole ripe peaches or 8 canned peach haves
½ cup almond or other cookie crumbs (amaretto cookies or almond macaroons are best, but you can substitute any nonchocolate cookie—even vanilla wafers will work, if you can't find fancier cookies or don't have time to make your own)
¼ teaspoon ground cinnamon
2 tablespoons chopped almonds
1 tablespoon amaretto liqueur or ¼ teaspoon almond extract (optional)
1 egg yolk
1 tablespoon sugar (optional)
Citrus peel or sliced almonds for garnish

Preheat the oven to 400 degrees.

Cut the peaches in half. Remove the pits and all traces of pits, then scoop out the centers so they are about the size of a tablespoon. Reserve any scooped pulp. Put the peaches, hollowed sides up, in a baking pan sprayed with nonstick cooking spray.

Combine scooped pulp, if any, with the cookie crumbs, cinnamon, almonds, liqueur or almond extract (if using), and egg yolk. Fill each peach with one-eighth of the mixture. Sprinkle the peaches lightly with sugar, if desired.

Bake about 20 minutes, until the peaches are tender and the filling is golden. Garnish with curls of citrus peel or sliced almonds (or both).

Makes 4 servings.

Nutritional information per serving: 420 calories, 14 grams total fat (3 grams saturated fat, 7 grams monounsaturated fat)

✒ CITRUS COMPOTE

Citrus trees adorned the Mediterranean long before they adorned the southern shores of the United States. Citrus fruits are available all year round but are particularly seasonal during the winter, making this dessert a refreshing fall, winter, or early spring finish to a warm, hearty meal. Served extra cold in chilled glass dishes, it is also a cooling summer dessert.

An alternative to bringing the lemon and lime to room temperature is to pierce each with a knife and microwave 30 seconds each to bring out the juice.

This recipe is too tart for some, hence the optional sugar. You may not want to use it if you like a good pucker!

2 medium tangerines
2 medium oranges

1 medium red grapefruit
1 medium lemon at room temperature
1 medium lime at room temperature
1 to 2 tablespoons sugar (optional)
Fresh coconut slivers or chopped almonds for garnish
   (optional)

Peel the tangerines, oranges, and grapefruit. Segment, and trim the white pith. (You don't have to cut it all off, as pith is loaded with fiber and phytochemicals. Too much pith adds a bitter taste, however.) Halve or quarter any segments that are larger than bite-sized. Remove any seeds with a sharp knife. Combine the segments in a large bowl.

Quarter the lemon and lime and squeeze over the citrus segments. Or, halve and use a citrus juicer to extract the juice, then drizzle over citrus segments.

If desired, sprinkle with sugar and mix gently. Chill at least 1 hour and serve cold.

Serve in glass bowls. Garnish with slivers of coconut or a sprinkling of chopped almonds, if desired.

Makes 4 to 6 servings, depending on appetites.

Nutritional information per serving (roughly): 145 calories, 0.4 grams total fat (0 grams saturated fat, 0 grams monounsaturated fat)

✤ QUESTIONS AND ANSWERS

✤ *Is fruit juice just as good as fruit?*

Generally, no. While fruit juice is a preferable substitute to beverages with higher refined-sugar contents such as cola, fruit juice—especially the kind you buy in the store—is fruit without the fiber and serving for serving contains a lot more calories than a piece of fruit. Whenever possible, choose the fruit over the juice. If you can't live without your juice, select the kinds that contain pulp. The fruit juice with pulp also may have retained more vitamins and phytochemicals than a highly processed juice. If you own a juicer, juicing your own fruits can be fun, and you can be assured the juice is fresh and wholesome—certainly a fresh and healthful alternative to a cocktail or after-dinner drink. However, when you clean the juicer of all that pulp, you'll see how much of the fruit you are throwing away.

ℬ Is it true that apples can keep other foods fresher and help other fruits ripen faster?

Apples do help. Put an apple in your bag of brown sugar to keep the sugar from drying out, and toss another in with your potatoes to keep them from sprouting. Baked goods stay moister in the company of an apple. Apples also make other fruit ripen faster. If you want to speed up the ripening of other fruit, put a few apples in the fruit bowl. If you want your other fruit to last longer, however, don't put apples in your fruit bowl.

ℬ What are other interesting ways to include fruit in the diet?

- Freeze green grapes and watermelon cubes to use as ice cubes in beverages or to eat on a hot summer day instead of sugary popsicles or high-fat ice cream.
- Toss dried fruit into a stir-fry.
- To jazz up plain brown rice, add a few raisins, chopped dried apricots, and walnuts.

- Whenever possible, add fresh fruit to your bowl of cereal.
- Dried fruit adds texture and flavor to hot cooked cereal. Also try stirring fresh blueberries into oatmeal.
- Whenever possible, add fresh fruit to your yogurt.
- Stir dried fruit, chopped apples, or chopped cherries into your next batch of homemade bread.
- Tired of peanut butter and jelly? Peanut butter and pear or even date sandwiches are more nutritious and far more delicious.
- As long as we are on the subject of peanut butter, don't miss the ultimate treat: peanut butter and ripe banana sandwiches!
- Add crisp apple slices to your turkey sandwich instead of cheese.
- Dried cherries add tang and interest to salads.
- Cranberry sauce isn't just for Thanksgiving. Make it with apple juice concentrate instead of sugar and serve alongside any meat or as a spread for bread or toast.

ℬ Which fruits can be cooked and which can't?

Don't cook melons. They lose their sweetness. The exception is cantaloupe, which is tasty sliced and very briefly grilled. Most other fruits can be cooked one way or another. Apples and pears are superb when baked in the oven (see the recipe on page 152), and also work well in breads, pies, and cakes, providing sweetness and tartness. Grilled bananas are a special treat. Berries of all types work well cooked for jam or jelly, in breads, pies, cakes, muffins, and cooked into sauces. Citrus fruits and juices are often used in baking and in cooking, as they are a good complement to many main dishes, meat or otherwise. One delicious way to prepare your Thanksgiving turkey or roasted chicken is to brush it with orange marmalade during the last hour of cooking, and baste it with orange juice during cooking.

Fruits with pits, like peaches, apricots, nectarines, and plums, make superb jam, cobblers, breads, cakes, puddings, and pies, and are also a delicious complement for meat or other main dishes. Try grilling peach and nectarine halves basted with citrus juice for a summer treat. Dried fruits are perfect for cooking. In addition to their use in breads and other baked goods, dried fruits are delicious cooked on their own terms. For a warm, satisfying breakfast on a cold morning, combine raisins with chopped dried apples, dried apricots, dried dates, walnuts, and a little fruit juice and warm on the stove until the fruit is plumped. Good morning!

℘ *This chapter makes fruit sound so great, but the fruit in the supermarket isn't anything like you describe. Why not?*

Perhaps one reason that Americans don't consume as much fruit as people in the traditional Mediterranean region is that the fruit available in American supermarkets is often of inferior quality. Picked before ripeness, shipped hundreds or even thousands of miles, heavily waxed and sprayed, much of the fruit in the American food supply isn't particularly tender, juicy, or flavorful.

How many times have you opened the produce drawer of your refrigerator only to find that your fruit has turned rotten, or that the peach that looks good on the outside is brown and hard on the inside? Fruit is delicate and doesn't respond well to rough handling, long-term storage, or transportation across an entire continent. However, knowing a little about fruit, how it ripens, how to choose the best pieces, how to store it, and what its nutritional star qualities are can make the difference between a fruit-poor diet and a diet loaded with nature's very own sweet treats. A few rules apply in general to most fruits:

- Wash fruit thoroughly and scrub with a good fruit or vegetable brush to remove pesticide residue, dirt, microorganisms, and so on. Too vigorous scrubbing can bruise delicate fruit, however, so be gentle. Buy organic fruit if it is available and affordable. If fruit is waxed, consider peeling. Wax is virtually impossible to scrub off and can trap undesirable substances. Even though the skins of many fruits (like apples) are heavy with nutrients and phytochemicals, their pesticide residues may prove to be worth foregoing the extra nutrients when children will consume the fruits.
- Don't scrub fruit with soap, which isn't meant to be eaten, either. Try a fruit and vegetable wash instead.
- The greater the variety of fruits you consume, the fewer of one type of pesticide residue you'll be subjected to, and you'll receive a wider range of nutrient and phytochemical benefits.
- Most fruit will last longer when refrigerated and will ripen faster at room temperature. To speed up ripening, store a couple of pieces of fruit in a brown paper bag and roll the bag shut. Keep at room temperature and turn the bag daily to promote even ripening. Check frequently because some fruits ripen very quickly this way. This

method works great for fruits with pits, like peaches, nectarines, plums, and apricots. It also works beautifully for unripe pears, and bananas ripen extra quickly this way.

- Fruits are delicate. Handle gently, store carefully, and check often for bruises, cuts, mold, soft spots, or rot. Don't eat the bad spots.
- Fruits soak up water, diluting their flavor and encouraging spoilage. Whenever possible, wash fruit just before eating it. However, if it means the difference between not eating fruit and washing it before you store it, wash, dry, then store, and enjoy at will straight from the fridge. We understand that convenience is often the determining factor!
- The potent antioxidants in citrus juices (lemon juice, orange juice, etc.) work their magic on cut fruit that tends to brown. When cutting fruit for a fruit salad or for cooking, sprinkle or brush with citrus juice to keep the fruit from turning dark.
- Dried fruits like raisins and currants are more tender and pleasant to eat if you let them plump up in a little water, wine, or fruit juice for at least ten minutes before serving or using in a recipe.

6: *The Grains, Legumes, Nuts, and Seeds of the Mediterranean*

If vegetables are the soul of traditional Mediterranean cuisine, grains, legumes, nuts, and seeds are the body. This food group constitutes the bulk of the traditional Mediterranean diet, and the many manifestations of grains, legumes, nuts, and seeds are delicious, comforting, fragrant, filling, and deeply satisfying.

Nothing distinguishes a Mediterranean kitchen more than the aroma of fresh-baked bread. Whether a dense round loaf of country bread from France or crispy Moroccan flatbread, whole-grain bread accompanies most Mediterranean meals in one form or another. Imagine steaming pots of pasta in shapes ranging from prodigious lasagna noodles and giant shells to rice-shaped orzo and the "little ears" called orecchiette to couscous, the grainlike pasta so common in African and Middle Eastern cuisine. The types of pasta are endless: spaghetti, linguine, fettuccine, penne, rigatoni, ziti, conchiglie, and fusilli, to name just a few.

Creamy risotto, a heavenly Italian rice concoction, may be flavored with any number of vegetables from artichokes to zucchini. Other rice dishes are prevalent as well: saffron-colored Spanish rice that is the one consistent ingredient in a Spanish paella, the classic Greek rice pilaf, and various combinations of rice with vegetables or seafood, baked in the oven or added to soup.

Porridgelike when fresh, crispy when chilled, sliced, and grilled, cornmeal-based polenta is an Italian specialty, as are gnocchi, little Italian dumplings made with flour and often potatoes. From the Middle Eastern shores of the Mediterranean comes bulgur wheat, cooked into pilafs or tabouli salad. And then there are pizzas, calzones, vegetable and meat pies, moussaka. Anybody hungry?

Grains sit at the base of the Mediterranean Diet Pyramid, which suggests eight or more servings of whole-grain breads, pasta, cereal, rice, bulgur, couscous, polenta, and others each day. One of the best ways to eat Mediterranean is to add more whole grains to your diet.

Grains of all types are made even heartier and more delectable with the addition of protein-rich legumes, nuts, and seeds: penne with white beans, rice with peas, chickpeas with bulgur wheat, spaghetti with walnut sauce. Legumes are a fixture all over the Mediterranean, often taking the place of meat as a main course and, even more often, serving to stretch very small amounts of meat to serve many. Legumes contain many vitamins (such as folacin) and minerals (such as selenium), are protein- and fiber-rich, and satisfying dressed with nothing more than a little olive oil and a splash of lemon juice. Their sizes, colors, and types are far too numerous to list here, but some of the more common Mediterranean legumes are white canellini beans, chickpeas (garbanzo beans), fava beans (broad beans), black beans, green and red lentils, tiny white haricot beans, red kidney beans, lima beans, and Egyptian ful beans.

Many cultures have used legumes for centuries as a primary protein source, and the Mediterranean region is no exception. The Mediterranean Diet Pyramid suggests at least two half-cup servings of legumes each day.

Nuts and seeds (technically, nuts are large seeds of fruits with hard husks, except for peanuts, which are actually legumes) are often used to add flavor and crunch to raw and cooked foods, whether part of an appetizer, such as almond paste mixed with chickpeas for hummus; a feature of the main meal, such as pasta with pesto rich with pine nuts; or sprinkled over stewed fruit for dessert. Nuts and seeds can add significant nutrients, phytochemicals, protein, and monounsaturated fats to a traditional Mediterranean-inspired diet. Although most nuts and seeds can be high in total fat, generally only 10 percent of this fat is saturated. Frequent nut and seed consumption has been linked to low rates of many chronic diseases such as certain cancers and heart disease. Despite many fears that eating these beneficial foods (especially nuts) will cause weight gain, recent studies have shown otherwise. Walnuts, almonds, hazelnuts (filberts), pine nuts (pignolia), pistachios (in the Middle East), and peanuts (technically a legume) are the nuts most common in the Mediterranean.

Mediterranean or not, all nuts and seeds, except for the coconut (which is high in saturated fat) can be added to a Mediterranean-inspired way of eating. Just be sure that the nuts and seeds you consume (whether in spreads, such as peanut butter, or in the "whole" form) are not packaged with added hydrogenated oils, which spells trans fatty acids. Other types of nuts and seeds include chestnuts, cashews, pecans, pumpkin seeds, sesame seeds, and sunflower seeds. The Mediterranean Diet Pyramid suggests that nuts and seeds be consumed daily in quantities of at least 1 ounce, depending on your individual caloric needs or allowances. Nuts and seeds, either plain or roasted without added oils and salt, make a wonderful and convenient snack food. A handful of nuts or seeds along with some whole-grain crackers (preferably, crackers that also do not contain hydrogenated oils) and perhaps some dried fruit—raisins, currants, dates, and so on—make a nutritious quick fix between meals.

Grains, legumes, nuts, and seeds are delicious and fill-ing sources of good nutrition in the true Mediterranean style. Let's talk about some of their more stellar nutri-tional—and in the case of fiber, nonnutritional—health benefits.

❧ FABULOUS FIBER

Fiber, that nonnutritive stuff that gives plants their shape and sturdiness, is a word for carbohydrates that the body doesn't digest. If it isn't nourishment, how is it helpful? Even without nourishing the body, fiber does plenty to facilitate good health. Fiber alone is sufficient justification to choose whole grains over refined because of its many benefits.

Fiber adds roughage to the diet—that noncaloric bulk that keeps the digestive and elimination systems running smoothly. New research suggests that fiber may also keep the body from digesting some of the fat and protein it consumes. The study, conducted by the United States Department of Agriculture Human Nutrition Research Center in Maryland, put people on diets with the same number of calories but with differing, and changing, fiber content. When fiber intake was higher, absorbed calories were lower, making fiber a great ally for attaining and keeping body weight within a desirable range.

Fiber seems to do more than its famed role of prevent-ing constipation. Studies have linked high fiber intakes to decrease of certain cancers, such as cancer of the colon and rectum. It also appears to help stabilize blood sugar in people with diabetes and improve high blood cholesterol levels by lowering the bad LDL cholesterol. Fiber is bulky, therefore filling. Therefore, a meal rich in fiber doesn't leave much room for high-fat foods.

Fiber isn't all the same, however. It comes in two types, and each type performs a specific function in the body. Soluble fiber, present in many fruits and vegetables, dissolves in water and forms a gellike substance in the body. It works in the body to lower cholesterol levels, particularly levels of LDL ("bad") cholesterol, by bonding with bile acids, which are made of cholesterol, and moving them quickly through the intestines and out of the body so that less cholesterol is absorbed into the blood. Types of soluble fiber include pectin, guar gum, oat gum, and psyllium, and these are the substances linked to decreased risk of heart disease and diabetes. Soluble fiber is the much-publicized type of fiber in oat bran, which is why oatmeal and other oat-based cereals are now heavily advertised as heart-disease preventives. However, oats are not the only source of soluble fiber. Other good sources include whole-grain bread, barley, kidney beans, pinto beans, navy beans, lentils, split peas, black-eyed peas, green peas, corn, prunes, pears, apples, and citrus fruits.

Insoluble fiber is sometimes easier to spot. It is, and looks like, roughage, and includes substances like cellulose and lignin. This is the fiber that gives plants their structure. One of the best sources is wheat bran.

Insoluble fiber doesn't dissolve in water. In the body, insoluble fiber expands because it soaks up water. It helps move waste through the body quickly and is the fiber that may decrease the risk of certain chronic diseases by minimizing the time potentially harmful substances spend in the colon.

While whole wheat–based products are among the richest sources of insoluble fiber, some fruits and vegetables contain insoluble fiber, too: most notably, dates, blueberries and blackberries, green peas, and lima beans.

Many foods contain both types of fiber, and many fiber-rich foods are low in fat and high in vitamins and minerals, making the benefits of fiber hard to isolate. One thing is clear, however: Fiber-rich foods are good for your health!

Yet, most Americans don't consume as much fiber as many health officials would like—in one survey, the national average totaled about 11 grams of fiber per day, not impressive next to the levels recommended by many health organizations. The American Heart Association, the American Cancer Society, and the American Dietetic Association recommend 25 to 35 grams of fiber per day for the maximum health benefit. Those who consume too little fiber may be putting themselves at risk for colon cancer, as well as constipation, hemorrhoids, high blood pressure, diabetes, obesity, and coronary heart disease, to name just a few of the conditions linked to low-fiber diets.

To get more fiber of both the insoluble and soluble types into your diet, follow the Mediterranean way of eating, choosing fiber-rich foods daily: whole grains in breads, pastas, and cereals; a variety of legumes, nuts, and seeds; and a variety of fresh raw fruits and vegetables.

ℬ B VITAMINS, HOMOCYSTEINE, AND YOUR HEART

While fruits and vegetables are rich in many vitamins and minerals, when it comes to many of the B vitamins, whole grains and legumes are even better sources. B vitamins are water-soluble vitamins that include thiamin (B$_1$), riboflavin (B$_2$), niacin, folacin, pantothenic acid, biotin, pyridoxine (B$_6$), and cobalamin (B$_{12}$). They perform many functions in the body, from helping the body turn carbohydrates, fats, and sugars into energy to making cells.

B vitamins may also help to protect against heart disease. Heart disease researchers have linked high levels of a substance called homocysteine in blood to higher risk of heart disease. Homocysteine is a chemical formed naturally in the body from a breakdown of amino acids from protein foods. Generally, homocysteine levels don't pose a problem in the body. They are kept within a safe range by the action of three of the B vitamins: folacin, B$_6$, and B$_{12}$. However, when homocysteine levels rise, the walls of the arteries become sticky, catching blood cholesterol and encouraging its accumulation along arterial walls. This accumulation can eventually result in artery blockage, restricting blood flow to the body, including to the heart and brain. One study suggested that 15 to 30 percent of all patients with artery blockages had too-high levels of homocysteine in their blood.

While the homocysteine–heart disease connection is still largely unexplored—for instance, no studies have linked purposefully lowered homocysteine levels to any decrease in heart disease risk—it may make sense for people already at risk for heart disease to have their homocysteine levels tested and to take steps to lower homocysteine levels over 12 micromoles per liter. (Talk to your doctor if you are concerned.)

It certainly makes sense to eat foods rich in B vitamins, like whole grains and legumes. These foods are good for your health in many ways, and are a great way to keep homocysteine levels in check for anyone, whether or not you are currently at risk for heart disease.

For those eating a Mediterranean-inspired diet, getting enough folacin, B_6, and B_{12} (the latter available mostly in animal foods—more on B_{12} in the next chapter) is easy. For those whose diets consist primarily of "junk food"— candy bars, sodas, chips, and the like—deficiencies of these essential nutrients are far more likely.

✃ THE PHYTOCHEMICALS OF GRAINS, LEGUMES, NUTS, AND SEEDS

Vegetables and fruits aren't the only phytochemical-rich elements of a healthy diet. Grains, legumes, nuts, and seeds are plant foods, too! Some of the phytochemical stars in this group include:

- **Phytosterols.** These cholesterol-lowering, anti-cancer phytochemicals are contained in many nuts and seeds, such as almonds, cashews, peanuts, sesame seeds, sunflower seeds. Phytosterols are also abundant in whole wheat and soybeans (again, not a "Mediterranean" legume, but one that can and should be included in a Mediterranean-inspired diet), as well as in some vegetables (such as corn) and vegetable oils.
- **Lignans (or phenolic lignans).** Abundant in whole grains and flaxseed (not a Mediterranean original, but well worth a mention in any discussion regarding chronic disease prevention), this powerful "phyto" or plant estrogen helps protect the prostate and breast from cancer. Lignans contain antioxidant properties, and can also be found in some berries and vegetables.
- **Flavonoids.** These plant phenolic compounds are featured in wine, tea, and many fruits and

vegetables, but they are also present in many
types of legumes and cereal grains.

- **Phytic Acid.** This compound is found in cereal
grains, including wild rice, nuts, and seeds, especially sesame seeds and soybeans. Some
researchers believe that it is phytic acid, not fiber,
that provides the anticancer effect of diets rich in
whole grains, nuts, and seeds. Phytic acid seems
to slow cancer formation and stabilize blood
sugar, cholesterol, and triglyceride levels.

- **Saponins.** These phytochemicals may keep cancer cells from multiplying as well as keep blood
sugar, cholesterol, and triglyceride levels in
check. While most vegetables and herbs contain
some saponins, beans and legumes are the richest
sources.

- **Resveratrol.** This phenolic fungicide that gives
wine its color and may contribute to wine's heart-
protective function is present in even greater concentrations in peanuts.

❦ GETTING THE WHOLE GRAIN

While grain-based foods aren't always made from the
whole grain (grains that have not been stripped of their
bran and germ), traditional Mediterranean foods, especially breads, are far more likely to be made from whole
grains than many of the grain products popular with
American consumers: white or "wheat" (but not "whole
wheat") breads, refined pastas, and white rice, not to
mention a host of specialty products made with refined
white flour: dinner rolls, packaged snack cakes, bagels,
English muffins, breakfast muffins, and other sweetened
baked goods. Even so-called "health foods" can be

deceiving: rice cakes, cereal bars, and "health" breads aren't always made from whole grains and are sometimes highly refined.

Grains are the fruits of grass plants, and grains contain three parts: the germ or seed, which contains protein and oil; the endosperm, containing carbohydrates and some protein; and the bran, or outer layer. Once upon a simpler time, people picked grains, ground them between stones to make flour, and that was that. When technology made the removal of the coarser bran and germ possible, a finer, whiter flour was the result. This white flour was nothing but the ground endosperm, and although the endosperm contains protein and carbohydrates, most of the vitamins, minerals, and fiber are contained in the bran and germ—those valuable parts of the grain people began to throw away.

In the 1940s, manufacturers began to restore some of the missing vitamins and minerals to refined grain products. This may seem like a roundabout way to get the goodness of grain products into your body, and indeed, it is. In the past few decades, people have begun to prefer the coarser, heavier, whole-grain products once again, as public understanding about nutrition grows. We now know that white bread, white flour, white rice, and other refined grain products lack the nutritional value of their whole-grain counterparts.

Scientists have also uncovered a whole host of health benefits from whole-grain consumption. Whole grains, which provide vitamins such as folacin and vitamin E; minerals such as selenium and magnesium; phytochemicals such as phytosterols and lignans; and fiber, have been implicated as strong allies in the fight against a number of chronic diseases. Some of these diseases include certain cancers, such as cancer of the colon and rectum, as well as heart disease.

Not too long ago, oats made headlines as protectors against heart disease. As a result, foods containing oats, whole oats, and whole oat flour began to flood the market with brightly colored labels claiming that eating these foods "may reduce heart disease risk." The Food and Drug Administration (FDA), a government "watch dog" that regulates health claims on food labels, researched these purported promises. In 1997, the FDA, after examining studies involving soluble fiber and heart disease, approved that foods rich in whole oats can be deemed as heart healthy, so long as they contain at least 0.75 grams of soluble fiber per serving (a daily intake of at least 3 grams of soluble fiber has been shown to lower high blood cholesterol levels). The labels must also be worded in a way that indicates the importance of a low saturated fat intake in addition to whole oats in the diet.

Whole oats are not the only grains associated with a reduced risk of heart disease. In a recent study from the University of Minnesota, women between the ages of fifty-five and sixty-nine who ate at least three servings of whole grains in general per day over a nine-year period were 30 percent less likely to die of a heart attack than women who ate less than one serving of whole grains per day.

What makes whole grains a heart-disease preventive? The answer isn't yet clear but probably involves a number of factors: more vitamins and minerals, more fiber, and more phytochemicals, including phenolic compounds like flavonoids and coumarins; glucarates, carotenoids, terpenes, phytic acid, and phytoestrogens.

The fiber in whole grains has disease-fighting properties, too. Diets rich in fiber have been linked to lower incidences of colon and rectal cancer, in particular. Scientists suspect that fiber fights cancer because it "dilutes" potentially carcinogenic substances in the colon with bulk, and it also moves these substances through the body more quickly, allowing the body less time to absorb them. (For more on fiber, see above.)

The good health of people living in the Mediterranean and eating a traditional Mediterranean diet is certainly due, in part, to the heavy consumption of whole grains. Mediterranean breads are typically (though not always) dense, hearty, and heavy, with the nutty, chewy texture of whole-grain wheat and other grains. Many other traditional Mediterranean ingredients, from the stone-ground cornmeal used to make Italian polenta to the fluffy millet that accompanies many northern-African meals, consist of grains never subjected to the refining process. Refining grain products does make them last longer, and makes them lower in fat. The germ, which contains oil, is removed so the grain will become rancid far less quickly (oil becomes rancid, or decomposes, relatively quickly, and will last longer when refrigerated and not exposed to light). However, the germ in whole grains is an important source of vitamin E and other important nutrients, and shouldn't be left out of the diet.

ℬ GO WITH THE GRAIN

While most whole grains have been used to some extent in the Mediterranean, some are more well known than others. Some of the most beloved and most nutritious grains in the traditional Mediterranean diet were wheat in its many forms, from the pale yellow, hard-wheat semolina used to make pasta to the hearty bulgur wheat used to make tabouli; stone-ground corn for polenta; and rice in its many forms, from arborio rice for risotto to yellow (from added saffron) Spanish rice.

These grains aren't the only choices today, however, as

food production makes grains from all over the world available in the United States. Eating a variety of grains is the best way to assure plenty of soluble and insoluble fiber, vitamins, minerals, and phytochemicals. The high-nutrient, high-fiber grains commonly available today include:

- **Amaranth.** This grain, revered by the ancient Aztecs, is widely available today. It is exceptionally high in protein, vitamins and minerals, and contains lysine, an amino acid many grains are missing. You can buy whole amaranth grains or find amaranth in grain products, such as breads and pastas. Amaranth makes a flavorful hot cereal or an interesting side dish when mixed with other grains, such as cornmeal.
- **Barley.** Many people have only encountered barley in its traditional American manifestation, as part of a beef and mushroom soup. Barley is delicious in many other forms as well, however, as a breakfast feature or dinner accompaniment, in soups, salads, or combined with other grains. Pearl barley is the refined barley. It keeps longer but has less nutritional value. Scotch or pot barley is more nutritious and contains fiber.
- **Buckwheat.** This grain is featured in the cuisines of many countries. Kasha, a traditional Russian form of buckwheat commonly available, may not be Mediterranean, but it is delicious, nutty, filling, and satisfying.
- **Cornmeal.** Stone-ground cornmeal is the whole-grain variety and it makes a fine, hearty polenta, that dish beloved in Italy and just as delicious in the United States today. The version popular in the southern United States is better known as

grits. Either way, the whole-grain cornmeal contains fiber and has lots of minerals and vitamins.

- **Millet.** This African grain is more often seen in this country in birdseed mixes, but why should we let the birds get all the great nutrition? Millet is delicious as a hot cereal or mixed with olive oil, garlic, and grated cheese as a hearty side dish to a main meal.

- **Oats.** Who doesn't love a warm bowl of oatmeal on a cold morning? Whole-grain oats are full of soluble fiber, and they taste delicious on their own or combined with other grains in baked goods. Process oatmeal in your blender to make oat flour and substitute it for half the wheat flour in baking. Limit the use of instant or "quick-cooking" oats, especially those that are preflavored, as they can be high in sodium and sugar.

- **Quinoa.** This traditional South American grain is high in protein and minerals, cooks quickly, and is a delicious substitute for rice or bulgur. Combined with nuts, it makes a hearty snack or alluring side dish.

- **Rice.** Brown rice is higher in fiber, vitamins, minerals, and phytochemicals than white rice. It has a nuttier, richer taste. White rice cooks more quickly and lasts longer in the pantry. Rice combines well with many foods: tomatoes, beans, vegetables, nuts, herbs and spices, seeds, even dried fruit. Spanish rice is highly spiced with tomatoes, green peppers, garlic, and hot pepper; paella, another Spanish dish, consists of rice flavored with chicken or other meat, tomatoes, legumes, vegetables, and sometimes shellfish. Risotto is an Italian dish in which rice—Italian rice like arborio or medium-grained rice work best—is cooked with oil, stock, white wine, and Parmesan cheese (there exist numerous variations) to create a rich, tender, creamy dinner course.

- **Wheat.** This most ubiquitous of grains is highly versatile and present in virtually every cuisine worldwide. Notably, wheat was originally a Mediterranean grain. Perfectly suited for making bread, wheat is also available in numerous other forms: wheat berries, cracked wheat, couscous and other semolina-based pastas, wheat germ, and bulgur wheat are a few. As mentioned previously, whole wheat contains the bran, germ, and endosperm and is full of vitamins, protein, minerals, phytochemicals, and fiber. Whenever possible, choose whole-wheat products to get the maximum benefit. Wheat is one of the most fiber-rich of the grains, so enjoy it often—something easy to do in the United States, where wheat dominates the grain market.

♭ FULL OF BEANS

Whether you love beans or fear them, they are undeniably a rich source of protein, fiber, minerals, vitamins like folate, and phytochemicals like flavonoids. Beans are just one type of legume, a category that also includes peas and lentils. For thousands of years all over the world, people have relied on legumes for survival. They are low in calories, high in nutrition, and much less expensive than meat. They are also delicious and extremely versatile, adding flavor and interest to an astounding variety of foods. (See the recipe section on page 182.)

Whether you prefer dry or canned, plain or fancy, try to include legumes in your daily diet or at the minimum, three times per week. Legumes come in many shapes and sizes. Follow package directions for cooking instructions. If you are a beginner and a bit bean-wary, order some bean-based dishes in restaurants first. You'll know a professional is preparing them. As you get more daring, try them in your own homemade soups, on salads, in casseroles, rolled in tortillas, tossed with stubby pasta, or mixed with rice.

Mediterranean or not, include a variety of legumes for a diet in the Mediterranean spirit, such as black beans, black-eyed peas, cannellini beans, chickpeas, cranberry beans, fava beans, flageolets, great northern beans, lentils, lima beans, navy beans, peas, pink beans, pinto beans, red kidney beans, red beans, and split peas.

✌ NUTS (AND SEEDS) TO YOU

Nuts and seeds are loaded with nutrition, and no healthy diet should be without them. High in fiber, phytochemicals, protein, vitamins, and minerals, these antioxidant-rich food sources are as healthy as any other Mediterranean featured plant food. How can that be when they are so high in fat? Again, it's not simply total fat, but saturated fat that needs to be limited as much as possible for a healthy heart. Nuts and seeds generally contain very low amounts of saturated fat (the exception being the coconut), leaving room for the heart-healthy monounsaturated fat and omega-3 fatty acids (a type of polyunsaturated fat) to principally dominate these foods. Monounsaturated fat, the fat featured in olive oil, tends to lower your LDL (bad) cholesterol without affecting your HDL (good) cholesterol levels, thereby keeping your total blood cholesterol levels in check and reducing your risk of heart disease. The omega-3s have also been linked to healthy hearts, as well as to a decreased risk of certain cancers and other diseases.

Recent studies have shown the beneficial effects of nut consumption in particular in the fight against heart disease. A highly regarded study from Boston's Brigham and Women's Hospital (BWH), called the Nurses Health Study, showed that "women who ate at least 5 ounces of nuts per week reduced their risk for coronary heart disease by 35 percent compared to women who ate less than 1 ounce per month." Similar results may soon appear for men from an equally famous study, the Physicians' Health Study (also based out of BWH in Boston). In the DELTA (Dietary Effects on Lipoproteins and Thrombogenic Activity) study, which was funded by the Heart, Lung, and Blood Institute, participants who ate a diet with nuts being a primary source of the total fat calories substantially lowered their bad LDL cholesterol levels when switching from a high-fat typical American diet to a lower-fat diet that was rich in nuts.

In addition to diseases of the heart (which include coronary heart disease and congestive heart failure), the healthy fat content of nuts and seeds, as well as the fiber, phytochemical, and antioxidants they contain, have many researchers looking at the role of these foods in decreasing the incidence of other chronic diseases, such as certain cancers (such as breast cancer), diabetes, stroke, and renal failure.

Unfortunately, many Americans avoid nuts and seeds, fearing that the fats in these nutritious foods will cause weight gain. Indeed, most nuts and seeds are sources of fat (as mentioned above), and therefore calories. But there have been many intriguing studies showing how frequent nut consumption will not necessarily lead to weight gain. In a large study involving more than 34,000 Seventh Day Adventists in California, those who ate nuts at least five times a week had lower body weights than the rest of the group. Another study looking at 508 people living in Reno, Nevada, also showed that frequent nut eaters kept their weights within a desirable range. While this does not suggest that eating nuts will keep us thin, it helps to support the argument that nut (as well as seed) consumption should not be feared as a one-way ticket to obesity. (Some study subjects actually lost weight after adding nuts to their diet.) Researchers speculated that those who eat nuts tend to be more conscious about their health. Those benefits of course were rendered from the "fresh" nut, or nuts that have not been processed in hydrogenated oils.

Indeed, eating any food to any large degree (especially if you don't substitute a certain food calorie for another) will cause weight gain. But although most nuts and seeds contain their fair share of fat and calories, they should not be condemned. If you follow the recommendations of this book, nut and seed consumption is listed in the daily food section in moderate amounts (to be adjusted for individual caloric needs). Meats, higher-fat dairy, and other high–saturated fat foods have been pushed farther up on the pyramid, to be consumed on a weekly or monthly (if at all) basis, all depending on their level of saturated fat. For many, these higher saturated fat foods will therefore be consumed less frequently, leaving calories to be replaced with nuts and seeds.

Confused? Let's look at the numbers. In an ounce of almonds, which is about twenty-four nuts, you've got roughly 165 calories. Alternatively, eat an ounce of potato chips, and you've comparably consumed about 155 calories. And which of these two foods is far more beneficial for your health? No question, the almonds! You may find that eating the almonds is a lot more satisfying than the chips, since the nuts contain a lot more fiber and feel more "wholesome" than the processed snack item. Hence, you may feel less compelled to keep on snacking, saving you even more calories in the long run. And some research has even indicated that the high fiber content found in nuts, as well as seeds, may prevent all of the calories and fat in nuts and seeds from being absorbed anyway.

For another example, let's look at a breakfast. Instead of eating an egg (which contains about 80 calories, 5.5 grams of total fat), mix about ½ ounce of almonds (about twelve nuts) into your whole-grain cereal for 83 calories, 7.5 grams of fat. The numbers compare, and tossing ready-made almonds into your cereal is a lot more convenient than having to cook an egg. You may also find you are more satisfied with the almonds. See the following Q & A for a list of common nuts and seeds, and their fat and calorie breakdown. Replacing nuts and seeds for other less healthy foods has been done in some controlled studies, with the results proving positive, especially, again in the realm of heart disease prevention. A study published in the *New England Journal of Medicine* in 1993 found that when walnuts replaced 20 percent of the calories in the diet of one group (the walnut diet was adjusted to include lesser amounts of other fatty foods), total cholesterol levels went down and LDL-HDL cholesterol ratios improved. The study concluded that "incorporating moderate quantities of walnuts into the recommended cholesterol-lowering diet while maintaining the intake of total dietary fat and calories decreases serum levels of total cholesterol and favorably modifies the lipoprotein profile in normal men." The walnut, incidentally, has been a part of the Mediterranean diet for thousands of years.

Whether the grains, legumes, nuts, and seeds you choose to form the bulk of your diet are those of the traditional Mediterranean or not, enjoy these most gratifying foods and reap their nutritional benefits daily. These foods are an endless source of interesting recipes and make filling, deeply satisfying comfort food.

The following are adapted from recipes provided by the Walnut Marketing Board in Sacramento, California, and The Bean Education and Awareness Network in Chicago, Illinois.

℘ RECIPES

⚜ SWEET CORN AND TOASTED WALNUT RISOTTO

½ cup chopped walnuts
1 large onion, chopped
2 large cloves garlic, minced
1½ cups uncooked arborio rice
Three 14½-ounce cans fat-free, reduced-sodium chicken broth
4 ears fresh sweet yellow corn, husked, silk removed, and kernels cut from cobs
Salt and freshly ground black pepper, to taste
½ cup chopped fresh chives
¼ cup nonfat grated Parmesan cheese

In a dry skillet over medium-high heat, heat the walnuts for 1 to 2 minutes until the walnuts are slightly toasted. Set aside.

Coat a 12-inch round nonstick skillet with vegetable cooking spray and set over medium-high heat. Add the onion and sauté, stirring occasionally for 3 minutes. Stir in the garlic; sauté for 1 minute. Add the rice and stir often until it turns opaque, about 2 minutes. Stirring constantly, add the chicken broth, half a can at a time, adding more broth only when the rice has absorbed the previous amount. When adding the last half-can broth, stir in the corn kernels. When the rice is tender, the risotto is creamy, and the corn is cooked, remove from heat. Stir in the walnuts. Season with salt and pepper. Divide the risotto among six warm individual serving bowls and sprinkle with chives and Parmesan cheese.

Makes 6 servings.

Nutritional information per serving (roughly): 388 calories, 3g fiber, 10 grams total fat, 1.5 grams saturated fat, 4.3 grams monounsaturated fat)

✒ TUSCAN BEAN SOUP

1 cup chopped onion
½ cup chopped celery
3 cloves garlic, minced
1 tablespoon extra-virgin olive oil
1 tablespoon flour
¾ to 1 teaspoon dried rosemary
¼ teaspoon dried thyme
2 bay leaves
1 whole clove
¼ teaspoon freshly ground black pepper
Four 14½-ounce cans reduced-sodium chicken broth
One 17-ounce can baby lima beans, rinsed and drained
One 15-ounce can garbanzo beans, rinsed and drained
One 15-ounce can red beans, rinsed and drained
2 tablespoons low-sodium tomato paste

1½ cups cooked barley
1 large potato, unpeeled, cut into ½-inch pieces
1 cup sliced carrots
1 cup packed sliced spinach leaves

In a large saucepan, sauté the onion, celery, and garlic in the oil 2 to 3 minutes; stir in the flour, herbs, clove, and pepper, and sauté until the onions are tender, 2 to 3 minutes longer. Add the chicken broth, beans, and tomato paste to the saucepan; heat to boiling. Reduce the heat and simmer, uncovered, 20 to 25 minutes, adding the barley, potato, carrots, and spinach during the last 10 minutes of cooking time. Discard the bay leaves and clove.
Makes 6 servings.

Nutritional information per serving: 335 calories, 5 grams total fat (.45 gram saturated fat, 1.2 grams monounsaturated fat)

✤ FALAFEL WITH TOMATO-CUCUMBER RELISH

One 15-ounce can garbanzo beans, rinsed and drained
1 medium onion, coarsely chopped
¼ cup packaged parsley leaves
2 cloves garlic, minced
½ teaspoon ground cumin
¾ teaspoon dried oregano
2 to 3 teaspoons fresh lemon juice
Salt and freshly ground black pepper to taste
1 cup dry whole wheat bread crumbs
¼ cup chopped raisins
1 egg yolk
Olive oil cooking spray
Tomato-Cucumber Relish (recipe follows)

In a food processor fitted with the metal blade, process the garbanzo beans, onion, parsley, garlic, cumin, and oregano until smooth; season to taste with the lemon juice, salt, and pepper. Stir in ½ cup of the bread crumbs, the raisins, and egg yolk.

Form the bean mixture into 16 patties using about 1½ tablespoons for each. Coat the patties with the remaining ½ cup bread crumbs.

Spray a large skillet with the cooking spray; heat over medium heat until hot. Cook the falafel patties over medium heat until browned on the bottom, 2 to 3 minutes. Spray the tops of the falafel with cooking spray and turn; cook until browned on the bottom, 2 to 3 minutes. Arrange 4 falafel on each plate; serve with the Tomato-Cucumber Relish.

Makes 4 servings.

Nutritional information per serving (4 falafel with Tomato-Cucumber Relish): 311 calories, 4 g fat, .5 g saturated fat, .9 gram monounsaturated fat, 54 mg cholesterol)

✐ TOMATO-CUCUMBER RELISH

½ cup chopped tomato
½ cup chopped cucumber
⅓ cup fat-free plain yogurt
½ teaspoon dried mint (optional)
Salt and freshly ground black pepper, to taste

In a small bowl, combine the tomato, cucumber, yogurt, and mint leaves; season to taste with salt and pepper.

🍃 FRENCH CASSOULET

1¼ pounds boneless, skinless chicken breast or pork
   tenderloin cut into ¾-inch pieces
12 ounces low-fat smoked sausage cut into ½-inch
   slices
1 tablespoon extra-virgin olive oil
1½ cups chopped onions
1 cup chopped red bell pepper
4 to 6 teaspoons minced garlic
Four 15-ounce cans great northern beans, drained
   and rinsed
One 14½-ounce can diced tomatoes with roasted garlic
1 teaspoon dried thyme
1¾ cups fat-free, reduced-sodium chicken broth
Salt and pepper, to taste
2½ cups fresh plain whole-wheat bread crumbs

Preheat the oven to 350 degrees.

In a Dutch oven, sauté the chicken and sausage in the
oil until lightly browned, 8 to 10 minutes. Add the
onions, bell pepper, and 3 to 5 teaspoons of the garlic;
cook over medium heat 5 minutes. Stir in the beans,
tomatoes, thyme, and chicken broth; season to taste with
salt and pepper. Put mixture into casserole pan.

Combine the bread crumbs and remaining garlic;
sprinkle over the top of the bean mixture. Bake uncovered until the crumbs are browned and the beans are
thickened, about 1½ hours.

Makes 8 servings.

*Nutritional information per serving (roughly): 485 calo-
ries, 7 grams total fat (1.8 grams saturated fat, 3.1 grams
monounsaturated fat, 60 mg cholesterol)*

✍ MOROCCAN VEGETABLE STEW

1 medium eggplant, unpeeled, cut into 1-inch cubes
6 small onions, cut into quarters
4 cloves garlic, minced
4 tablespoons olive oil
1 teaspoon ground cinnamon
¾ teaspoon ground cumin
¼ teaspoon ground turmeric
¼ teaspoon ground cloves
⅛ to ¼ teaspoon cayenne pepper
¼ teaspoon freshly ground black pepper
3 cups chopped seeded tomatoes
3 medium zucchini, sliced
2 medium sweet potatoes, cut into ¾-inch pieces
1 green bell pepper, cut into ¾-inch pieces
1 cup sliced celery
One 15-ounce can chickpeas, rinsed and drained
One 15-ounce can red kidney beans, rinsed and drained
½ cup reduced-sodium chicken broth
2 tablespoons minced parsley

In a Dutch oven or large saucepan, sauté the eggplant, onions, and garlic in 2 tablespoons of the oil 3 to 4 minutes over medium heat, or until the eggplant is beginning to brown. Stir in the seasonings; cook 2 minutes longer.

Add the remaining ingredients except the parsley to the Dutch oven. Heat to boiling; reduce the heat and simmer, covered, until the vegetables are tender, 10 to 15 minutes. Stir in the parsley.

Makes 6 to 8 servings.

Nutritional information per serving (roughly): 340 calories, 12 grams total fat (5.14 grams saturated fat, 6.07 grams monounsaturated fat)

🌾 BASQUE PAELLA

1 cup chopped onion
3 tablespoons extra-virgin olive oil
1 cup long- or medium-grain rice
2 cloves garlic, pressed
1 teaspoon ground cumin
One 15-ounce can whole tomatoes, halved (do not drain)
One 13¾-ounce can reduced-sodium chicken broth
1 cup dried tomato halves, cut into strips with kitchen shears
12 ounces shelled shrimp, deveined (with or without tails)
One 15-ounce can pinto beans, rinsed and drained, or 1½ cups cooked pinto beans
One can (15 ounces) light red kidney beans, rinsed and drained, or 1½ cups cooked light red beans
1 cup diced trimmed zucchini (¼ inch pieces)
1 cup fresh, frozen, or canned corn kernels
Salt to taste
¼ cup chopped fresh cilantro
2 tablespoons finely chopped red bell pepper
1 teaspoon finely chopped, seeded jalapeño pepper

In a 12-inch skillet over medium heat, sauté the onion in the oil about 5 minutes, until golden. Add the rice, garlic, and cumin; reduce the heat to low and stir 1 minute. Add the canned tomatoes with their juice, the broth, and dried tomatoes; heat to boiling, stirring once. Cover; cook over medium-low heat 15 minutes.

Meanwhile, in a bowl, mix the shrimp, beans, zucchini, and corn. Add to the skillet and stir to mix. Cover and cook over low heat about 10 to 15 minutes, depending on the size of the shrimp, mixing often until the shrimp is opaque throughout. Season with salt.

Transfer the paella to a serving dish. Sprinkle with the cilantro, bell pepper, and jalapeño just before serving.

Makes 6 main-course servings.

Nutritional information per serving: 440 calories, 10 grams total fat (1.24 grams saturated fat, 5.4 grams monounsaturated fat, 110 mg cholesterol)

🌿 MEDITERRANEAN VEGETABLE AND WALNUT SALAD WITH OLIVE VINAIGRETTE

½ cup chopped walnuts
½ cup prepared reduced-fat balsamic vinaigrette dressing
1 tablespoon minced, pitted ripe olives
One 15½-ounce can no-salt-added chickpeas
1 medium red bell pepper, seeded and thinly sliced
1 large carrot, peeled and cut into matchsticks
1 small red onion, thinly sliced
4 cups each spinach and arugula leaves

In a dry skillet over medium-high heat, heat the walnuts 1 to 2 minutes until they are slightly toasted. Set aside.

In a small bowl, whisk together the vinaigrette and olives. Set aside.

In a medium bowl, combine the chickpeas, bell pepper, carrot, and onion; toss with 3 tablespoons of the vinaigrette and olives. Set aside and reserve.

In a large bowl, toss the spinach and arugula with the remaining vinaigrette; divide equally among six salad plates. Top with the vegetable mixture and sprinkle with walnuts.

Makes 6 servings.

Nutritional information per serving (roughly): 381 calories, 10 grams total fat (1 gram saturated fat, 4.5 grams monounsaturated fat)

✸ QUESTIONS AND ANSWERS

✸ *Fresh whole-grain bread sounds great, but I don't have time to make it at home. Any suggestions?*

Many bakeries and even grocery stores bake delicious whole-grain breads that can be purchased fresh each day. Also, consider buying a bread machine. These machines make homemade bread a breeze, and they have the added benefit of filling your home with the aroma of baking bread. Just pour in the ingredients, press a button, and the machine does the rest. Fresh bread in a few hours!

When time does permit—a free weekend afternoon, for example—try baking your own bread by hand. Few things are more relaxing and rejuvenating than mixing, stirring, kneading, pounding down, kneading again, forming, and baking your own bread. Good exercise, too!

✸ *What if I don't like whole-grain products?*

Like olive oil, whole-grain products can be an acquired taste, especially if you are accustomed to refined-grain products. Whole-wheat bread is usually an easy switch. It is more flavorful with a more interesting texture than white bread. Whole-grain pastas, tortillas, and cereals are a harder sell for some, although others like them immediately.

Don't worry about transforming every single grain product in your diet to whole grain, especially right away.

Make the steps gradually. The more you become acquainted with the interesting flavors and textures of different whole grains, the more willing to experiment you may become. But don't force yourself to eat something you don't like. Maybe for now, only white spaghetti will do, but perhaps you don't mind the nutty flavor of brown rice. Just keep an open mind. Eventually you may find yourself purchasing buckwheat groats for breakfast, sprouted wheat pita bread stuffed with falafel for lunch, and amaranth vermicelli for dinner!

ℬ *What are additional ways to get more fiber into my diet?*

One convenient way for Americans to add fiber to their diets is to eat a serving of whole-grain cereal every morning. If you like hot cereal, choose old-fashioned or steel-cut oats rather than instant. When purchasing cold cereals, check the labels and choose varieties with higher fiber content. If you are a toast lover, choose from the wide variety of delicious whole-grain breads (preferably those that do not contain hydrogenated oils). Make pancakes or waffles with whole wheat or oat flour for a change.

For lunch, choose whole-grain bread for your sandwich, or toss some beans or chickpeas and a handful of sunflower seeds onto your salad. Choose a bean-based soup with rice or pasta.

For dinner, choose brown rice over white, and experiment with different types of whole-grain pasta. Whenever possible, eat your fruits and veggies raw and chew them well (chopping and cooking can modify the fiber content of some foods). Wash produce well so you needn't discard the edible peels, often rich sources of fiber. Substitute beans in your meal for meat at least twice a week, and begin replacing half the white flour in cooking and baking with whole-wheat or other whole-grain flour. And don't forget to snack on popcorn, nuts, and seeds, all good fiber sources.

✤ How much fiber is required for a food to be labeled "high fiber"?

The nutritional information on packaged food will list that food's fiber content. However, any food labeled "high fiber" must contain at least 5 grams of fiber per serving. If the label says a food is a "good source" of fiber, that food must contain between 2.5 and 4.9 grams of fiber per serving. "More fiber" or "added fiber" means the food contains at least 2.5 grams per serving *more* than a serving of the traditional version of that food. Remember, the goal is to consume about 25 to 35 grams of total fiber per day.

✤ Will too much fiber cause digestive problems?

A sudden increase in fiber intake can cause temporary digestive problems such as flatulence and stomach cramps. Instead, increase your fiber intake gradually, giving your body a chance to adjust. First switch to whole-wheat bread. A week later, choose a whole-grain cereal. A week after that, add more raw vegetables. And so on.

Legumes are notorious for their gas-producing quality. However, discarding the water in which you've soaked dried beans and cooking the beans in fresh water can significantly lower the gas-producing effect of beans. If you prefer the convenience of canned beans, rinse them well before cooking and eating (this step will also minimize the high sodium content of some canned beans). For some, smaller portions take care of the problem.

If you do notice unpleasant digestive effects from an increased fiber intake, cut back just a little until your body doesn't seem to notice, then increase again, gradually. If you are willing simply to ride out the effects, they won't last long. Once your body adjusts to your healthier, fiber-rich diet, you shouldn't notice any ill effects. For painful gas problems, several over-the-counter remedies are available (but if pain persists, please see your doctor).

Exceptionally high intake of fiber (over 50 to 60 grams daily) has been shown to cause serious intestinal problems when the fiber is taken as a supplement rather than received through the consumption of natural, whole-grain foods like bread, pasta, and cereal. We recommend you receive your fiber through your diet, not through supplements, fiber powders, or fiber pills. Also, people with certain digestive diseases may need to limit fiber intake or consume fiber in specific ways. If fiber is a problem for you because of a health problem, contact a registered dietitian to help you work fiber into your diet.

℘ What is the best way to soak dried beans for cooking?

To minimize gas content, soak dried beans in room-temperature water in a large container (the beans will approximately triple in size) for at least four hours, or put them in soaking water before you go to bed at night, then cook them the next day. When you are ready to cook them, drain off the soaking water and boil them in fresh water until they are fork-tender. Don't add salt or any acidic foods like vinegar or tomato products until the very end of cooking time. These will hinder the beans from becoming tender. A dash of olive oil will keep the bean water from foaming.

If you don't have time to soak the beans for four hours and cook for another few, boil water, remove from the heat, and soak the beans in the hot water for one to four hours, then cook. Or use canned beans. They are as nutritious as dry beans, although they are typically softer and, some say, less flavorful. Rinse canned beans well before use.

ℬ Are garbanzo beans and chickpeas the same thing?

Yes.

ℬ What is the fat and caloric content of commonly eaten nuts and seeds?

While most nuts and seeds contain their fair share of fat, and therefore calories, the fat that they contain is principally the beneficial monounsaturated kind. Nuts and seeds also contain omega-3 fatty acids. Both monounsaturated fat and omega-3 fatty acids have been shown to help guard against many chronic diseases, such as heart disease and cancer.

The chestnut is one nut that is actually a low-fat food. In an ounce of roasted European chestnuts (which is about three and a half nuts), there is only *0.6 grams* of total fat, *0.1 grams* of saturated fat, and 70 calories. The chestnut is definitely a food that should be indulged in (within reason, of course) during the holidays, or beyond, if you can find them in your local market.

Other popular types of nuts and seeds with their fat and calorie content are noted below.

Nut or Seed (1-ounce serving)	Total Fat (g)	Saturated Fat (g)	Calories
Almonds (24)	15	1	165
Cashews, dry roasted (about 18)	13	2.6	165
Chestnut, European, roasted (3½)	0.6	0.1	70
Peanuts, dry roasted (about 36)	14	2	160
Pecans, dried (31 large)	19	1.5	190
Pistachios, dried (47)	14	1.5	165
Sesame seeds, whole, toasted	13.5	2	160
Sunflower seeds/ kernels, dried	14	1.5	160

Note in the above chart that an ounce of most nuts and seeds can actually be quite plentiful. For example, 1 ounce of peanuts is thirty-six nuts, 1 ounce of pecans is thirty-one large, and 1 ounce of pistachios is 47 nuts. Sitting down and eating this many nuts at once can be a challenge for many. Hence, eating more than the above calories from this food group is probably unlikely. The Mediterranean Way Pyramid recommends eating a variety of nuts and seeds to be consumed throughout the day to equal about 1 ounce or so daily. Another way of getting nuts is through nut spreads such as peanut butter or almond butter that do not contain added hydrogenated oils (which translates as trans fatty acids), sugars, or other fillers. Two tablespoons of a nut spread equals 1 ounce.

7: *Meat, Poultry, Fish, Dairy, and Egg Consumption the Mediterranean Way*

The chapter that might, in many books about dietary considerations, be a book's centerpiece is put nearly last in this book—not because we don't like meat and dairy products, but because they were, in comparison to plant foods, of so little importance in the traditional Mediterranean diet. That's not to say people in the Mediterranean don't eat meat. They always have, and many of the most well known and beloved Mediterranean recipes contain meat. However, the traditional Mediterranean diet is a near-vegetarian diet.

Near vegetarian? The term may sound contradictory, but in a culture accustomed to a large slab of beef on the center of a dinner plate surrounded by a few paltry servings of vegetables, the term makes sense. In the traditional Mediterranean diet, beef, as well as veal, pork, fish, poultry, and rich dairy products like cheese, was more often used for flavoring rather than as the main event of a meal.

Nestled in a large platter of rice and vegetables, one might find a few small pieces of chicken or shrimp. A prodigious pot of pasta sauce might contain a few clams, some prosciutto, or perhaps some ground meat. Occasionally a whole fish poached with vegetables and herbs will form the core of a meal, and various types of shellfish are present in small quantities in the diets of most Mediterranean countries. A Turkish or Greek shish kebab typically includes cubes of skewered lamb, but plenty of vegetables, too.

Eating some meat and dairy products certainly makes good sense. High in nutrients, including certain vitamins and minerals, meat and dairy products also add depth, dimension, and flavor to plant foods. Even red meat can be a sensible part of a healthy diet, if the cuts of meat are lean. Yet, because high-fat meat and full-fat dairy products contain high amounts of saturated fat, they are best included in small amounts. Eating these foods in moderation is ideal because it guarantees you the nutritional benefits of these animal foods without the excess saturated fat, not to mention excess calories. Pushing animal foods to the side of the plate leaves room for the highly beneficial plant foods we've been discussing throughout this book.

The Mediterranean Diet Pyramid illustrates how animal foods can fit into a healthful Mediterranean-inspired diet. In addition to fish (weekly consumption is recommended), you can choose a serving of another source of lean meat about once a week, if desired. Serving sizes are specified in a general range of 1 to 4 ounces on the Mediterranean Diet Pyramid, to be individualized according to dietary needs. Remember, you needn't consume your entire week's allowance of fish, lean beef, chicken, veal, or whatever you choose at one sitting. An ounce chopped and added to soup one day, another ounce or two added to rice or pasta a few days later, and a few more ounces in a casserole at the end of the week is probably a more authentically Mediterranean way to eat animal foods anyway. The same goes for cheese—a few shreds here, a sprinkling there. A little high-fat cheese, which is highly flavored, goes a long way. Although the Mediterranean Diet Pyramid specifies lower-fat cheeses (such as mozzarella made with part-skim milk) be consumed optionally on a weekly basis or high-fat cheese be consumed monthly (also optional), that month's serving can easily be portioned out over a number of satisfying meals.

Try to choose the animal products listed closer to the base of the pyramid more often than those listed higher— fish more than chicken, chicken more than lean beef, and so on. These animal meats are arranged by their saturated fat content; the farther up they are listed, the more saturated fat they contain. The same goes for dairy products: High-fat dairy products, such as high-fat cheeses, butter, and so on, sit at the top of the pyramid, while lower-fat cheeses are listed within the weekly section. (We placed the "lower-fat" cheeses as an optional weekly treat because cheese was very much a part of the traditional Mediterranean cuisine, albeit usually in smaller amounts per serving than typically seen in the United States today). Low-fat or nonfat dairy products are listed in the daily echelon of the Mediterranean Diet Pyramid—a great way to keep your daily protein and calcium intake at a satisfactory level.

Fish is the one animal meat we recommend consuming more often—up to 8 ounces of cooked fish per week— especially, believe it or not, the fattier fishes like salmon, mackerel, trout, herring, and tuna. Fish contains omega-3 fatty acids that offer many health benefits (more on omega-3 fatty acids later in this chapter).

And what about eggs, those high-cholesterol villains we all know to avoid? Actually, before, dietary cholesterol isn't a threat to the heart health of most people.

There are indeed some who are particularly sensitive to dietary cholesterol, usually a genetic condition. Consult your physician if you think this might be you. It is saturated fat, as we've mentioned throughout this book, that has been clearly linked to a higher risk of heart disease. Egg yolks do contain some saturated fat, which is the main reason why we generally suggest a moderate intake of four or fewer eggs per week (including eggs used in cooking). By the way, the egg white is virtually cholesterol- and fat-free, so indulge at will on this high-protein portion of the egg.

ℬ THE VEGETARIAN MEDITERRANEAN

Typically, the traditional Mediterranean was not a land of vegetarians. But what if you aren't particularly fond of meat, or eggs, or even dairy products? Perhaps you are a vegetarian and don't think the Mediterranean Diet Pyramid could be relevant for you. Please don't read our recommendations for animal products as a requirement. You needn't eat meat or eggs at all, especially if you are diligent about following the recommendations in the "daily" section of the Mediterranean Diet Pyramid. This level contains no meat or eggs. While a little animal meat or egg can go a long way, nutritionally speaking, and while fish certainly has demonstrated health benefits, none are a necessity in a healthy diet.

Probably the question vegetarians hear the most is: "How do you get enough protein?" You may have even thought the same thing when surveying the Mediterranean Diet Pyramid. Meat just once a week? How could that be enough? What about protein?

Actually, most Americans consume much more protein than their bodies need—about 90 grams of protein each day, mostly from meat and processed meat. The average man typically needs about 60 grams of protein per day, the average woman about 50 grams. Because saturated fat can be high in animal food sources, plant-based protein sources, although often less protein-dense, may be a healthier protein source. Getting enough protein takes little effort for the average adult (pregnant and breastfeeding women need slightly more). Breakfast alone can knock off a third or more of this requirement: ¾ cup of oatmeal (dry) mixed with 1½ cups of nonfat milk (to be cooked), then topped with ½ ounce of nuts and a cup of strawberries comes to about 25 grams of protein.

Come lunchtime, a green salad with 1 tablespoon sunflower seeds and ½ cup garbanzo beans, 2 cups of hearty lentil soup, a whole-wheat roll, and a cup of nonfat plain yogurt mixed with fresh fruit comes to about 25 grams. For dinner, try 2 cups whole-wheat pasta topped with mushrooms, artichoke hearts, broccoli, green and red peppers, tomato sauce (with Italian seasonings), ½ cup white beans, and 1 tablespoon of Parmesan cheese; with a baked apple, the protein adds up to about 35 grams (or more, depending on the amount of vegetables—cooked vegetables, contain roughly 3 grams of protein per ½ cup). This meal rounds out the total to a more than satisfactory 85 grams of protein. And what do you know—no meat!

Of course, that's just one day, and if you were to be true to the traditional Mediterranean diet, meat would eventually enter the picture, albeit in small amounts, here and there, as flavoring. While we wouldn't discourage you from eating vegetarian, this book is about the eating patterns of the traditional Mediterranean region, and these include a wide and fascinating variety of plant foods, as well as animal foods in small quantities sufficient to provide enough protein for the entire family. We won't dispute that animal foods offer the most complete source of protein, meaning they include all the amino acids our bodies need. However, protein-rich plant foods in abundance and in a wide variety can do a great job of meeting our amino acid requirements as well.

If, however, you prefer to go completely without meat, eggs, and fish, you could be at risk for a vitamin B_{12} deficiency. Without enough vitamin B_{12}, you could develop a severe blood disorder called pernicious anemia. Vitamin B_{12} is found mostly in foods of animal origin, most notably in certain fish, such as clams, mackerel, tuna, and shrimp, as well as beef and lamb. Milk and dairy products also contain some vitamin B_{12}, as well as certain fortified cereals (check the labels). If you consume no foods of animal origin whatsoever, we recommend consultation with a dietitian or other qualified health care professional to ensure adequate vitamin B_{12} intakes.

Strict vegetarians may also have difficulty getting enough vitamin B_6 into their diets. The highest sources of this vitamin are certain fish such as bass and salmon. Certain plant foods are also rich in vitamin B_6. If you don't eat meat or fish, be sure to include in your weekly consumption those plant foods containing vitamin B_6, such as chickpeas (garbanzo beans), whole grains, potatoes, bananas, avocados, and dried figs. Again, consultation with a registered dietitian or other qualified health professional would be beneficial for those strict vegetarians.

Minerals that may be deficient without the consumption of animal protein include zinc and iron. Meat, poultry, and fish are good sources of zinc, but so are whole grains and certain vegetables.

Iron is an essential mineral. Without it, people can develop an iron-deficiency anemia. People experiencing rapid growth stages—children, teenagers, menstruating and pregnant women—are especially in need of iron in their diets.

Iron comes in two forms: heme iron and nonheme iron. Heme iron is found only in animal meats and egg yolks. Nonheme iron is found primarily in plant foods such as whole grains, seeds, nuts, greens, legumes, and dried fruits. Nonheme iron is much less efficiently absorbed. However, the absorption of nonheme iron can be improved when combined with vitamin C or animal food sources containing heme iron.

Although our body needs iron, consuming amounts far above the recommended daily allowance can be dangerous. Some researchers believe that excessive iron intakes can lead to heart disease, or even cancer, especially in those who are not in need of a lot of iron, such as adult men. The heart disease–iron theory was fueled by results of a 1992 study involving more than two thousand adult males in Finland. The study showed that those men with the highest levels of iron in their blood were more than twice as likely to experience a heart attack as the men with lower levels. There has since been more recent research disputing this claim, but many experts still believe that iron fortification of foods such as bread products should be stopped because of the possible health risks for people who are not in need of large amounts of iron. For now, however, consuming animal meats in moderate amounts will help keep iron, especially the easily absorbable heme iron, at more reasonable levels. For more information on iron, contact your local registered dietitian or other health-care professional.

Vegetarian considerations aside, for those who choose to eat in a manner as close as possible to the traditional Mediterranean diet, foods of animal origin do help to ensure prevention of vitamin and mineral deficiencies. Of course, anyone with special nutrient needs, such as children, teenagers, pregnant women, and lactating women can benefit from the advice of a registered dietitian to assure they are meeting their unique nutritional requirements.

The key is to remember that the traditional Mediterranean diet remains staunchly plant-based and the ratio of plant foods to animal foods appears to be exceptionally conducive to good health and longevity. While many aspects of the traditional Mediterranean diet have been implicated in its apparent healthful quality, low animal product consumption may be a significant key to the health benefits of the traditional Mediterranean diet.

Let's look more closely at how these foods fit into a cuisine that cherishes yet hardly relies on them for nutritional support, and how you can mirror the Mediterranean pattern of animal food consumption in your own life by centering your diet around plant foods, then flavoring it with animal foods. Your heart will thank you, and your grocery bill will be lower too!

❧ MEDITERRANEAN MEAT AND POULTRY

The people in the Mediterranean like to eat meat. Make no bones about it! However, as much as they have always relished meat, people living around the Mediterranean Sea and eating a traditional Mediterranean diet simply don't eat much of it. Meat was expensive and hard to come by. A Mediterranean farmer was likely to have a few chickens and rabbits running around the farmyard, but cattle for beef? Mediterranean diet researcher Ancel Keys may have put it best: "Cows do not thrive where the olive tree flourishes—and vice versa!"

The Mediterranean landscape is particularly unsuited to grazing cattle into adulthood. The required pastureland simply isn't there, so the Mediterranean doesn't produce much dairy or beef cattle. Instead, cattle are slaughtered when young (veal) and, not inconsequentially, far lower in fat. In the traditional Mediterranean diet, veal, as well as lamb, were more common offerings than beef.

But even veal and lamb aren't present at every meal. What an expense that would be! In contrast, in the United States, beef is the most beloved meat (although red meat consumption has declined in recent years). Pork and chicken are also extremely popular.

Poultry and game were also a part of the traditional Mediterranean diet, but again, quantities were small and a meal centered around poultry was rare. Wild rabbits and wild game birds such as wild geese and ducks, pheasant, and quail often provided flavoring for the soup pot. Game tends to be lower in fat than domesticated animal meat (see the Q&A section for more on game meat). Wild rabbit is low in fat, with only 3 grams of fat per 3-ounce cooked serving. Domesticated rabbits can be high in fat, however—up to 8 grams of fat per 3-ounce cooked serving.

When meat is prepared as the center of a meal in the Mediterranean, it is often because of a holiday or celebration. Veal shanks braised with vegetables and served with risotto comprises the much beloved dish the Italians call osso bucco. Roast lamb, whether sliced and highly spiced or skewered and marinated, is the ultimate treat in Greece as well as in other Mediterranean countries such as Morocco.

In many other well-known Mediterranean dishes, meat enhances but doesn't dominate the flavor. Ground lamb flavors many Greek dishes such as moussaka or the stuffed grape leaves called dolmathes. Meatballs and other appetizers made with chorizo sausage are popular in Spain. Sausages of all flavors and containing different types of meat are available in most Mediterranean countries but are eaten in small quantities—their high salt and spice content made them a good way to preserve meat in the warm Mediterranean climate. Simmered with fava beans, sliced and baked with eggs and tomatoes, chopped and tossed into paella, dense and highly seasoned handmade sausages give many Mediterranean dishes their distinctive character.

Even when meat dominates a Mediterranean recipe, it is well surrounded by plant foods of all types. All the Mediterranean countries include meat, poultry, and seafood in their own versions of stews, soups, and casseroles, but these same dishes are brimming with juicy, fresh vegetables and tender grains. Meat is cooked with vegetables, roasted with olives, served alongside pasta, pilafs, and couscous, or variously sliced, skewered, ground, chopped, or cubed into salads. Meat can be found in risotto, legume-based baked dishes, mounds of fresh steaming pasta, or fancifully crafted appetizers, from Italian antipasti to Moroccan meze, that are as beautiful to behold as they are delicious to eat.

One last note about meat and the food pyramids we have discussed throughout this book: You may have noticed that the USDA food guide pyramid includes fish, legumes, eggs, and nuts in the "meat" group. The Mediterranean Diet Pyramid doesn't. Instead, we suggest that lean meat, poultry, eggs, and fish be consumed weekly, while nuts, seeds, and legumes be consumed daily. Meat's higher fat and cholesterol content make it a better occasional choice—a weekly treat, or a semi-weekly flavoring element for plant foods. With daily plant protein sources—legumes, nuts, seeds—you get the added benefits of fiber and phytochemicals.

ℰ PHASING OUT MEAT MAIN-COURSE MENTALITY

Much as you would like to eat a more plant-based diet, you may find it difficult to do. The United States is firmly entrenched in meat main-course mentality. Many of us retain that deep-down feeling that meat simply must be an important part of a healthy diet. Restaurants cater to this impulse by serving primarily meat-based entrées (although this is slowly changing, especially in ethnic and gourmet restaurants or restaurants with a health-conscious philosophy). When some restaurants do serve a meatless entrée, drowning the entrée's grains or vegetables in high-fat cheese sauces or mounds of melted shredded cheese often "compensates" for the lack of meat (as if a creative use of plant foods required any compensation). Striving to eat in the Mediterranean style certainly doesn't mean shunning animal products for the rest of your life. On the contrary, it means including a wide variety of animal products in your diet, but decreasing their importance and frequency of occurrence on your plate.

Shifting to a plant-based diet isn't difficult, it just takes a little creativity. You may also find it easier to limit your consumption of meat if you know meat isn't forbidden. You can still enjoy meat (meaning beef, pork, veal, lamb, and poultry—we'll talk about fish separately) while you focus on an enjoyment and exploration of plant foods as your primary dietary objective. Following are some tips to help you gradually shift that focus, while shifting that piece of meat to the perimeter of your plate:

1. Begin planning your meals for the week. If you don't plan, you may be more likely to fall

back on habit and rely on convenience or fast foods, much of which can be high in fatty meats. Planning ahead allows you to shop sensibly and it also cuts down on the hassle of trying to figure out what to make each night when everyone is hungry and wants to eat five minutes ago.

2. When planning, begin by allowing for four or five meals per week that include some meat (this can be further decreased later), but only one where meat is the center focus—for instance, a pork roast or sirloin steaks. Other choices could include meat but not emphasize it. Instead of beef burritos, use half the meat and stuff those tortillas with nonfat refried beans. Instead of fried chicken, chop some chicken and stir it, along with plenty of chopped vegetables, into yellow rice.

3. Each week, choose one piece of meat from the meat department and consider it a challenge to your creativity to make the meat last all week. You'll be more inclined to use small amounts in order to make the meat last. A roast can be served with potatoes and salad one night, and leftovers can be cooked into rice, tossed with pasta, shredded over salad, and stirred into soup for the rest of the week. A little goes a long way. A package of lean ground beef or some skinless chicken breast can easily last all week when they make up a small component of the main course.

4. After a few weeks, you can begin to reduce the amount of meat in recipes even more. Aim for red meat as a flavoring element in a recipe once a week, poultry on another night, and fish on

another night or two. Many Mediterranean-inspired recipes are conducive to such an effort. A Spanish paella varies from cook to cook in the Mediterranean, so why not experiment with your own versions? A few ounces of cooked chicken or lean turkey sausage and a few pieces of fish or chopped shrimp flavor a huge pot of yellow rice and vegetables. Sauce for pasta, eggplant moussaka, or other casseroles need contain no more than a few ounces of ground meat. Just a handful of any type of chopped meat is enough to enrich a soup brimming with vegetables and potatoes or pasta.

5. Experiment with substituting seafood where you would normally use meat or poultry. Shrimp, chunks of fish, or scallops are delicious with rice, stir-fried with vegetables, or tossed into a pot of soup. A grilled or baked (not deep fat–fried!) fish sandwich is a tasty alternative to the pervasive American cheeseburger, and cooked shrimp or crab adds flavor and interest to salads.

6. Keep experimenting with nonmeat dinners like pastas with sautéed vegetables, rice casseroles, vegetable pizzas and calzones, flavored polentas and risotto, and salads of all types—chopped vegetable salad, bread salad, rice salad, bean salad, bulgur salad, lentil salad, pasta salad, lightly dressed greens and citrus fruits, tomato salad with olive oil and feta cheese—the possibilities are endless.

7. Buy most of your groceries from the produce sections of your supermarket aisles. Eventually you may not even notice those brightly lit bins of cellophane-wrapped meat.

8. Get in the habit of shopping at farmer's markets or local produce stands when possible, stopping at the supermarket for staples only.

9. Finally, reserve the large pieces of roasted meat for holidays and special occasions. Turkey is a great low-fat food when eaten in moderation without the skin. The white meat is the lowest in fat. If your holiday traditions include a beef roast, pork roast, roast lamb, or even a roast goose, you will still be eating in the Mediterranean spirit, where roasted meats were cherished as a feature of special celebrations. Have a small portion, enjoy it, and load up on the plant-based side dishes.

10. Once you start to eat in a more plant-centered mode, you may find you don't miss meat much at all. At least, we've found this to be true in our own experience. A meal full of interesting plant-based dishes can be much more fun and interesting to eat than a plate of meat.

❧ THE BOUNTIFUL MEDITERRANEAN SEA

Seafood, in contrast to meat, has been and continues to be far more popular in the Mediterranean than in the United States. Certainly, part of this has to do with the omnipresence of the Mediterranean Sea. Fish, especially small fish, and shellfish were readily available, fresh, and inexpensive. Of course they would represent a major source of protein for Mediterranean countries.

Every Mediterranean country uses seafood pervasively in its cuisine. Fish soup alone is a feature of almost every Mediterranean country: Called *zarzuela de pescado* in Spain, *soupe de poissons* in France, *Cioppino* in Italy, and *Psarosoupa* in Greece, all typically contain, along with a variety of fish, plenty of vegetables and a dash of olive oil. Baked fish is a feature of the Mediterranean as well, and each country has its additional seafood specialties. Along the Mediterranean coast of Spain, paella, studded with shellfish such as shrimp, scallops, and mussels is a tradition and one of the hallmarks of Spanish cuisine. In France, bouillabaisse is the definitive seafood stew. Shellfish such as scallops cooked in olive oil and lightly dressed in a butter-garlic sauce are a delicacy, and a perfectly poached fish is a matter of pride in a French kitchen.

In Italy, risotto is often flavored with clams, shrimp, or squid. Swordfish may be served with pine nuts and dried fruit or baked with capers and olives. In the Middle East, fish may be served with any number of highly flavored sauces. Greek meals may begin with an appetizer of marinated octopus, and the main meal is more likely to include fish, often baked with vegetables and flavored with olive oil and lemons, than meat. Fish stuffed with spiced rice and baked or flavored with a seasoned charmoula marinade then skewered and grilled is a coastal Moroccan specialty.

In the United States, however, especially in the landlocked center, really good, fresh fish is much harder to come by, and many of the types of fish common in the Mediterranean are virtually unheard of in this country. However, we have many fresh fish and shellfish species of our own. The fresher, the better and more Mediterranean in character. One need not eat a native Mediterranean fish to eat in the Mediterranean style. Many easily available fish and shellfish species work well in traditional Mediterranean recipes.

Try salmon, snapper, haddock, halibut, or cod in the seafood recipes on pages 188 and 227 or your favorite recipes. The lobsters, crab, mussels, and shrimp may be of a different variety in this country than they are in the markets of France, but so what? As we've said many times before, substituting what is locally available and fresh is perfectly compatible with Mediterranean style. Or, forget the recipes and go for simplicity: bake, poach, steam, or grill your fish or shellfish with a little olive oil, then serve with a wedge of lemon.

Americans have no excuse not to eat more fish. Fish is, in general, a low-fat food, but even the high-fat types of fish, such as salmon, contain a type of highly beneficial fatty acids called omega-3 fatty acids. These fats are most prevalent in fish that frequent the chilly ocean depths. Consumption of salmon, albacore tuna, sardines, mackerel, herring, and bluefish has been linked to lowered heart attack risk.

✇ HEART-HEALTHY OMEGA-3s

The link between fatty fish consumption and lowered risk of heart disease was first well publicized in the late 1970s, when researchers discovered that the Greenland Eskimos, whose diets were heavy in fish, had extremely low levels of coronary heart disease. Omega-3 fatty acids seem to keep blood from clotting easily and accumulating on artery walls, and may even keep artery walls from hardening. Omega-3 fatty acids also appear to keep the heart pumping on a regular rhythm. (If the rhythm is disrupted, medically termed *arrthymia*, a fatal heart attack can occur.) These actions have been linked to lower incidence of heart disease and heart attacks.

The relationship between high consumption of omega-3 fatty acids and lowered heart attack risk didn't end with the Greenland Eskimos. Many studies since have reinforced the theory that fish is good for your heart. One study demonstrated how omega-3s may be even more beneficial to people who have already suffered a heart attack. In a recent study reported in the *Tufts University Health & Nutrition Letter*, men who had previously suffered a heart attack and were told to eat more fatty fish were 30 percent less likely to die during a two-year period than heart attack victims not told to eat fish. After two years, the fish-eating group had about one fifth the cardiac deaths as the other group, and only one third as many nonfatal heart attacks. Another study, detailed in the *Nutrition Action Newsletter*, found a 29 percent decrease in overall death during a two-year period in men who ate fatty fish twice each week. Additionally, studies show that fish oil may address cardiac arrhythmia, or irregular heartbeats, by stabilizing the heart's muscle cells. Laboratory studies showed that omega-3 fatty acids kept myocardial cells from losing calcium, a mineral they require for normal operation. And other studies have demonstrated time and again that people who eat as little as one meal of fatty fish a week (usually salmon) suffer about half the cardiac arrests as those who don't regularly eat fatty fish.

Fish isn't the only source of omega-3 fatty acids—vegetarians who don't eat fish can benefit, too. A type of omega-3 called alpha-linolenic acid is found in some plant foods and has also been linked to lower heart attack risk. Sources of alpha-linolenic acid include certain vegetable oils (most notably flaxseed oil, canola oil, and in lesser amounts, olive oil), walnuts, soybeans, and other beans. Traces of this omega-3 fatty acid can also be found in kale, wheat germ, avocados, strawberries, and broccoli. In one study, women who ate the most alpha-linolenic acid were about half as likely to die of a heart attack as women who ate the least amounts. Those who had the lowest risk of dying from a heart attack consumed about 1.4 grams of alpha-linolenic acid daily, the equivalent of about a tablespoon of canola oil, 1⅓ table-spoons soy oil, or a cup of olive oil (too much olive oil to consume daily, of course—canola oil is probably the most practical and widely available source).

It is easy to see how the omega-3s can promote heart health, considering their effect on blood coagulation. Omega-3 fatty acids make blood less sticky and likely to clump up and clog arteries, as well as less likely to form blood clots. Yet, they have been shown to benefit more than the heart.

ℬ OMEGA-3s FOR TOTAL HEALTH

Omega-3 fatty acids have been extensively studied, and the results are in: omega-3s do more than help your heart to stay healthy. Research supports the theories that omega-3 fatty acids may help to prevent certain cancers such as breast cancer, ease arthritis pain, assist in infant development, treat depression, promote improved blood glucose control in type 2 diabetics, and even maintain healthy bones.

Omega-3s for cancer defense? Epidemiological stud-ies have shown that populations that tend to eat a lot more fish than typical Americans have fewer incidences of breast cancer. It may be that omega-3 fatty acids help pre-vent the production of tumors in breast tissue, as some animal studies have indicated.

Clinical studies involving humans have yet to confirm whether omega-3 fatty acids prevent or cure breast can-cer, but some studies have determined that omega-3 fatty acids do tend to settle in the breast, and because of this, these fatty acids may play an important role in maintain-ing normal breast tissue. In a recent study at the University of California at Los Angeles, women with breast cancer were placed on a low-fat diet consisting of 3 grams of omega-3s each day, which equates to about 6 ounces of fatty fish. After three months, the amount of omega-3 fatty acids present in their breast tissue was significantly higher than before the study. Another study showed that malnourished cancer patients with advanced solid tumors consuming 18 grams of fish oil each day along with 200 IU of vitamin E lived longer and demonstrated improved immune function. Even though these preliminary human studies involved large intakes of omega-3 fatty acids, amounts that are not easy to maintain on a daily basis, the results are interesting. Definite proof of the correlation between omega-3s and cancer is still unknown.

Omega-3 fatty acids appear to help with inflammatory diseases. One such disease, and one that affects millions, is arthritis. In a recent ten-year study, arthritis patients consuming large doses of omega-3s experienced less joint swelling, tenderness, and morning stiffness. Many of these patients were able to reduce their intake of anti-inflammatory drugs, and some were able to get off anti-inflammatories altogether. The use of omega-3 fatty acids in the treatment of arthritis is still being determined, but there does seem to be some promise.

Another inflammatory disease that has received some attention from researchers involved with omega-3 fatty acid is cystic fibrosis. Feeding mice large doses of docosahexaenoic acid, or DHA (a type of omega-3 fatty acid found in fish), reversed the signs of cystic fibrosis. Human trials are underway.

DHA happens to be one of the chief fatty acids in the brain, and a substance developing fetuses get from their mothers in the last three months of pregnancy, when brain growth is most significant. For premature babies who miss that last trimester in the womb and are put on formula (rather than breast milk, which contains DHA), lack of maternal DHA may result in compromised brain, central nervous system, and visual development.

Even full-term infants fed breast milk appear to have enhanced brain development. Breastfed infants have scored higher on intelligence tests than those infants who were given formula without DHA. Whether these differences remained once the children reach school age has yet to be determined. But the apparent health benefits of DHA has lead many countries to start adding it to baby formulas, whether for premature or full-term infants. The same may be seen here in the United States, as the U.S. Food and Drug Administration continues to evaluate the scientific research for safe and effective baby formula fortification with DHA.

In keeping with the traditional Mediterranean way, we strongly recommend breastfeeding when possible to ensure your infant receives adequate amounts of DHA, as well as the many other benefits of breast milk. After all, traditionally women in Mediterranean countries primarily breastfed, and some speculate that this may be another reason for the low incidences of cancer in Mediterranean countries.

Preliminary research with omega-3 fatty acids has also shown promise for the treatment of depression. The rate of depression in the United States is on the rise. Today, more than 15 million Americans suffer from depression, and some researchers believe this increase is inversely proportional to the decrease in fish consumption in this country. Serotonin, a mood elevator in the brain, may not work as well in a less fluid environment, something the brain uses omega-3s to accomplish. While the link between fish oil and depression is still largely unstudied, it is interesting and worthy of further research.

Increased omega-3 fatty acid consumption may also help type 2 diabetics with improved blood sugar control. Population studies have shown that people who eat about 5 ounces of fatty fish each week appear to enjoy more controlled levels of glucose, as long as calorie intake is held constant. Substituting fish for other higher-fat meat sources (instead of simply increasing fish consumption) is advised. Excessive calories from any food can cause weight gain, and this can interfere with adequate blood glucose control. You thought only bones needed calcium? New animal studies suggest that omega-3 supports bone formation and could help to prevent or slow osteoporosis. There may come a day when dietary recommendations for osteoporosis prevention will include food sources of omega-3s, in addition to calcium.

✷ FABULOUS FISH

While many of the studies on the health benefits of omega-3s utilized fish oil supplements, side effects from too many supplements can be unpleasant—upset stomach, nausea, diarrhea, flatulence, weight gain, and the possibility of vitamin A and D toxicity and liver damage. No such side effects have been found from eating more fish, however. We should note that it appears that large amounts of fatty fish need to be consumed to reap most of the benefits listed in the above studies, but the jury is still out on how much we actually need. For now, why not eat more of this nutritious food in moderate amounts as recommended by the Mediterranean Diet Pyramid? Fish cooks quickly, making it a convenient choice for dinner, and it is versatile, fitting into many recipes as a meat replacement or featured on its own with nothing more than a little olive oil and fresh lemon juice. Fish with fins, such as flounder, cod, haddock, and catfish, are particularly low in saturated fat and cholesterol, and shellfish, although higher in cholesterol than fin fish, is also exceptionally low in saturated fat, the real concern when it comes to heart health.

Despite occasional warnings that tuna may have high levels of mercury and should be avoided by pregnant women and by children, or that seafood of various types may contain this or that toxin, in general, up to 6 to 8 cooked ounces of fish every week should be safe and, indeed, beneficial to health. Just to be safe, we don't recommend exceeding 8 ounces weekly for pregnant and lactating women, and suggest avoiding larger fish, like swordfish, which are higher on the food chain and more likely to be concentrated sources of any toxin. If you're concerned, consult your doctor, or pediatrician, about how much fish you and your children should be eating.

Despite the small risks, fish remains an excellent source of nutrition and is certainly in the spirit of the traditional Mediterranean diet—low in fat and great for heart health. Eat fish! But remember, moderate consumption is the most true to the dietary patterns of the traditional Mediterranean.

�456 THE IMPORTANCE OF DAIRY

While dairy foods didn't constitute a large part of the traditional Mediterranean diet, they were certainly important. Milk wasn't consumed in the quantities it is enjoyed in the United States. Reserved usually for coffee and custard, milk didn't keep well in the hot Mediterranean climate. Yogurt and cheese, however, lasted longer because of their fermented character, and while never dominating a meal, these dairy products certainly supported many a Mediterranean feast.

Dairy products from the traditional Mediterranean came from goats, sheep, buffaloes, and camels, as well as cows, giving Mediterranean cheeses much of their unique character. Yet, once again, dairy foods made up a relatively small portion of the traditional Mediterranean diet, and the health of the people eating this diet may reflect why low dairy consumption is best.

Yet, dairy products are a good source of calcium, and studies say Americans don't get enough calcium—most people should get 1,000 to 1,500 milligrams per day. Calcium appears to prevent osteoporosis, a bone-weakening disease affecting more than 28 million Americans, 80 percent of whom are women. Vitamin D added to milk helps the body absorb calcium more effectively. On the other hand, the fat content found in high-fat dairy products leaves less room for bone-strengthening calcium. Hence, the lower-fat dairy food varieties tend to be better sources of calcium.

Studies support the health benefits of dairy products for children, adolescents, and pregnant women—peak bone mass is achieved between the ages of twenty and thirty—so high calcium intake and high activity levels are crucial for children and youth up to this age. For those over sixty, when bone mass declines significantly, adequate calcium, coupled with adequate vitamin D intake, is also important.

High dairy calcium intake is thought to reduce the risk of osteoporosis and fractures, as well as colon cancer

and high blood pressure. However, excessive animal protein intakes have been found to cause calcium loss,
thereby increasing your risk of heart disease. High-fat
dairy products have also been linked to an increased risk
of coronary heart disease. During his international
explorations of diet and heart disease, Ancel Keys found
that people in Finland, where coronary heart disease
rates are among the highest in the world, ate exceptionally high amounts of dairy products and milk. Saturated
dairy fat was probably the culprit.

Although people living in the Mediterranean countries
traditionally did not consume a lot of dairy, they probably consumed plenty of calcium from plant foods like
dark green vegetables. (Note: some green vegetables,
such as kale, contain calcium that is highly absorbable,
but some other green vegetables, such as spinach, contain
calcium that is not readily absorbed by the body. Eat a
variety of different dark green vegetables, and you will
probably get good calcium absorption from this plant
food category.) Other good plant sources of calcium
include figs, sesame seeds, almonds, tofu (when processed
with calcium salts—not a part of the traditional Mediterranean diet, but certainly a food that should be included
in the Mediterranean Way diet plan), orange juice (especially those varieties that are fortified with calcium),
white beans and other beans. These foods, of course,
have not been linked with increased coronary heart disease risk.

So what is a dairy lover to do? Dairy products are,
undoubtedly, a good source of calcium. In low or nonfat
form and in moderation, they are great dietary choices. If
you live for cheese, couldn't give up your fruit-flavored
cup of yogurt, or require warm milk before bedtime,
stick with low- or nonfat dairy products in moderation,

with two servings (or more depending on different individual needs) per day as specified in the Mediterranean Way Pyramid (a serving equals a cup of low-fat or nonfat milk or yogurt or 1 ounce of low-fat cheese). Some cheeses that are not considered to be low fat but are generally lower in fat than other cheese varieties can also be enjoyed in moderation on a weekly basis. These types of cheeses include part-skim mozzarella, part-skim ricotta, and reduced-fat feta (see page 232 for more on the fat content of selected cheeses). We've included these lower-fat cheeses in the weekly section because of their importance in flavoring many Mediterranean-inspired dishes. What would a homemade pizza be (preferably one loaded with a variety of vegetables for the ultimate Mediterranean treat) without a bit of part-skim mozzarella on top? Some researchers even believe the saturated fat in yogurt and cheese may not have as detrimental an effect on blood cholesterol levels as the saturated fat in butter and milk, although more studies on this are warranted.

℘ CHEESE, YOGURT, AND MILK

Cheese (as mentioned above) has been an essential component of Mediterranean cuisine for millennia. No dietary element could be more Mediterranean. As early as 4000 B.C., descriptions of cheese were recorded on clay tablets by the ancient Sumerians. Egyptian hieroglyphics depict cheese, and cheese was well known in ancient Greece and Rome.

Even today, cheese is a Mediterranean fixture. Italy alone has some sixty kinds of cheese and greater than three hundred cheese names that identify the locality of production. Spain is the exception when it comes to the Mediterranean love affair with cheese. Spanish cuisine isn't much concerned with cheese. In the other countries around the Mediterranean Sea, however, cheese was and is indispensable.

European cheeses are gaining in popularity in this country. Sales of feta cheese rose by 12 percent between 1995 and 1996. Sales of edam cheese rose 32 percent and asiago 21 percent. Even so, for years the American cheese "ideal" was a far cry from cheese in the traditional Mediterranean diet. As much as Americans love cheese, the cheese most familiar to us—big orange blocks of cheddar or chunks of Swiss, individually wrapped cheese sticks or sandwich slices, or that stuff known enigmatically as "cheese food"—would be strange and possibly frightening to a resident of the traditional Mediterranean.

Americans tend to prefer their cheeses mild and melted in large quantities over burgers, nacho chips, and Americanized versions of Italian food. This wasn't the way cheese was consumed in the traditional Mediterranean diet. A small cube of finely crafted hard cheese was often a dinner finale. When used in cooking, hard cheeses like Parmesan and Romano were grated lightly over or sliced and mixed in with vegetables. Softer cheeses like mozzarella were served in small amounts with tomatoes or marinated vegetables. A small chunk of feta is traditionally crumbled into Greek salads. Creamy cheeses would sometimes flavor or be stuffed inside vegetables or pasta in amounts just enough to impart a cheesy flavor without overwhelming the goodness of the principal components, the plant foods.

When it comes to cheese, the nutritional trick is to eat it in small amounts. Many cheeses are high in fat and sodium. Eating cheese in the Mediterranean style means eating cheese in small amounts, and usually choosing lower-fat varieties such as mozzarella (genuine mozzarella is made from Indian buffalo milk, but the version in the United States is made from cow's milk), low-fat ricotta, or reduced-fat feta (made from goat's milk). When high-fat cheeses are appropriate for certain dishes, a little goes a long way in the traditional Mediterranean diet. Strongly flavored cheeses accentuated the taste of food rather than drowning it.

Low-fat cheese can certainly be a part of a healthy daily diet. The Mediterranean Diet Pyramid recommends that nonfat or low-fat dairy products like low-fat cheese be consumed daily. Lower-fat cheeses (such as part-skim mozzarella) can be enjoyed on a moderate, weekly basis. Save high-fat cheeses for special occasions or consume them in very small amounts.

Yogurt has enjoyed similar popularity in the traditional Mediterranean diet, most notably in Greece and the Middle East, but also in other Mediterranean countries. When made with nonfat or low-fat milk, yogurt is an excellent part of a daily diet. It is low in fat, high in calcium and protein, and rich with the bacteria that can help maintain intestinal flora.

Milk was a far less popular part of the traditional Mediterranean diet than of the American diet. As we've mentioned, the warm climate and lack of refrigeration made cheese and yogurt the more practical and long-lasting dairy products. As Americans happily guzzle milk into adulthood, people in the traditional Mediterranean typically drank milk only with their morning coffee or espresso. As long as milk is nonfat or low-fat and consumed in moderation, it is an excellent source of calcium and other nutrients. The Mediterranean Diet Pyramid suggests nonfat or low-fat dairy products like skim milk be a part of the daily diet because of their high calcium and nutrient content.

✿ EGGS

What Spain lacks in cheese cuisine, it makes up for in its heavy use of eggs, making eggs a peripheral but important part of the traditional Mediterranean diet, at least as the Spanish have always known it. During his travels through Spain, Ancel Keys discovered that along the Mediterranean coast of Spain, eggs are eaten "at almost every main meal" while heart attacks remain a rarity compared to levels in the United States, and blood cholesterol levels of people living in this region were much lower than average levels in the United States. Keys attributes this seeming paradox to the fact that dietary cholesterol is less significant for heart health than saturated fat, and that despite high egg consumption, total saturated fat consumption remained low.

Eggs?! Aren't they little packages of dietary cholesterol just waiting to induce heart attacks in their unsuspecting victims? One large egg yolk (the whites don't contain cholesterol) has about 260 milligrams of dietary cholesterol, and the American Heart Association recommends a total daily intake of only 300 milligrams of cholesterol at most. One egg almost meets an entire day's quota! But, as we've said before, cholesterol really isn't a factor in heart health when consumed in moderation. Saturated fat is the dietary component to watch, and while eggs have some (one large egg also has about 6 grams of fat, of which about 30 percent is saturated), four eggs or fewer per week are fine for most adults. (Check with your doctor if you are unsure about whether you should be eating eggs.)

Moderate egg intake—that is, four or less per week as specified in the Mediterranean Diet Pyramid—is compatible with most of the dietary patterns seen in the traditional Mediterranean countries. It also just happens to be within the range recommended by the American Heart Association for people trying to prevent high blood cholesterol or treat blood cholesterol that is already moderately high.

✤ RECIPES

While the Mediterranean recipes you may often see in cookbooks will feature meat, we have tried to include those recipes that include it for flavoring but do not emphasize it, as we feel this is a more accurate reflection of how most people actually eat in the traditional Mediterranean.

✦ SPAGHETTI WITH MEAT SAUCE

When it comes to spaghetti, a little ground meat goes a long way. A sauce rich with vegetables and tangy tomatoes needs only a little meat to add depth and richness to its flavor.

Some Italian meat sauces, such as those from Bologna, have a higher proportion of meat to sauce and also add bacon and chicken livers. However, according to Ancel Keys, the people in Bologna had significantly higher blood cholesterol levels than the Italian people living along the coast of the Mediterranean. We prefer to keep the meat content, and our blood cholesterol levels, a little bit lower!

1 medium onion, chopped
2 cloves garlic, minced
2 medium carrots, scraped and shredded
1 small stalk of celery, finely chopped
3 tablespoons extra-virgin olive oil
¼ pound extra-lean ground beef
One 28-ounce can tomatoes with juice pureed in a blender or food processor (it can be chunky, but it should look like sauce)
2 tablespoons tomato paste
2 tablespoons chopped fresh Italian (flat-leaf) parsley
1 bay leaf
½ cup dry red wine (optional)
1 pound spaghetti, linguine, or vermicelli
Fresh grated Parmesan cheese (optional)

In a large saucepan over medium heat, sauté the onions, garlic, carrots, and celery in the olive oil. When the onions are translucent but not brown, add the ground beef. Break up the meat with a wooden spoon and cook until brown. Stir in the tomato puree, tomato paste, Italian parsley, bay leaf, and the wine, if you are using it. Reduce the heat and simmer about 30 minutes, until thick but not dry. (If the sauce gets too dry, add a little broth or water.)

In the meantime, cook the pasta in boiling salted water according to the package directions, until al dente (tender but firm—if you overcook pasta, it gets mushy). Drain the water and return the pasta to the warm pan (do not return to the hot burner). Just before serving, add the sauce and toss well. Pass fresh grated Parmesan cheese for those who want it.

Makes 6 to 8 servings.

Nutritional information (roughly): 385 calories, 8.5 grams total fat (1.5 grams saturated fat, 5.5 grams monounsaturated fat)

🌿 SEAFOOD RISOTTO

10 large shrimp, peeled and cut into bite-sized pieces
½ pound crabmeat or lobster meat, cut into small chunks
½ cup extra-virgin olive oil
3 cloves garlic, minced
1 cup minced onion
1 carrot stalk, peeled and chopped
1 medium stalk of celery, minced
½ cup finely chopped red bell pepper
½ cup finely chopped green bell pepper
6 cups water or broth
2 cups uncooked arborio rice or medium-grain white rice
½ cup chopped fresh Italian (flat-leaf) parsley
¼ cup freshly grated Parmesan cheese

In a large saucepan over medium heat, gently sauté the seafood in the olive oil. Stir about 5 minutes. Remove the seafood (but not the oil) and set aside. Add the garlic, onion, carrot, celery, and bell peppers to the oil. Sauté the vegetables until they are tender but not brown.

In the meantime, set the water or broth on the stove to simmer.

Add the raw rice to the oil-vegetable mixture and mix to coat the rice with the oil, fully incorporating the vegetables. Then, begin to add the simmering broth, a ½ cup at a time, letting each addition become almost completely absorbed by the rice and vegetables before adding the next ½ cup. When the rice is tender and saucy-looking, stop adding broth (even if you haven't added it all) and stir in the cooked seafood.

Remove from the heat and stir in the Italian parsley and Parmesan cheese. Serve immediately.

Makes 6 to 8 servings.

Nutritional information per serving (roughly): 285 calories, 17 grams total fat (3 grams saturated fat, 12 grams monounsaturated fat)

✒ SOUPA AVGOLEMONO

This famous Greek egg-and-lemon soup is a perennial favorite. Avgolemono as a sauce is delicious over meat or vegetables, but as a soup, it is elegant, deeply satisfying, and easy to prepare.

6 cups chicken broth
¼ cup short-grain rice
1 tablespoon each water and cornstarch
3 large eggs
3 tablespoons fresh lemon juice
1 tablespoon chopped fresh Italian (flat-leaf) parsley
Salt and freshly ground black pepper to taste

In a medium saucepan, bring the chicken broth to a boil. Add the rice and allow to boil for about 20 minutes, or until the rice is cooked. Reduce the heat and allow to simmer gently (not boiling).

Meanwhile, combine the cornstarch with the water, stirring until dissolved. Set aside. In a small bowl, beat the eggs until light, whisk in the lemon juice, and stir in the cornstarch/water mixture. Quickly whisk in ¼ cup of the hot stock. Add the egg mixture to the simmering stock, stirring briskly and constantly about 2 minutes until the soup thickens slightly. Stir in the parsley, season with salt and pepper to taste, and serve immediately.

Serves 8.

FOR THE TOTAL RECIPE: 87 calories, 5 grams total fat, (1.4 grams saturated fat, .75 grams monounsaturated fat.)

🌿 EGGPLANT PARMESAN

A delicious, filling, meatless meal, Eggplant Parmesan is quintessentially Italian and is a good example of how the Italians use cheese. This dish is at its best when the eggplant is cooked quickly to absorb the least amount of oil and the ingredients are fresh.

1 small onion, finely chopped
2 cloves garlic, minced
¾ cup extra-virgin olive oil
One 28-ounce can diced tomatoes
2 medium firm and fresh eggplants (weighing about 1 pound each)
½ cup flour
2 large eggs, beaten lightly
1 cup dried bread crumbs, flavor of choice, whole-grain preferable
1 pound part-skim mozzarella cheese
1 cup freshly grated Parmesan cheese
1 tablespoon chopped fresh Italian (flat-leaf) parsley

Preheat the oven to 400 degrees.
Prepare the tomato sauce: In a medium skillet over

medium heat, sauté the onion and garlic in ¼ cup of the olive oil until the onion is translucent but not brown. Add the diced tomatoes and stir to combine. Simmer gently 15 to 20 minutes, until the sauce thickens slightly. Remove from heat.

Meanwhile, wash and slice the eggplants into thin slices (¼ inch thick at most). (You can peel it if you prefer, but it isn't necessary.) Dip the eggplant slices in the flour, then into the egg mixture, then into the bread crumbs to coat. In a large skillet, heat the remaining ½ cup olive oil until a bread crumb sizzles on contact. Fry the eggplant slices quickly and carefully until tender, adding more oil if necessary. Drain on paper towels on a wire rack and salt lightly.

Slice the mozzarella cheese into thin slices.

Coat a 9 × 13-inch baking pan with ½ cup of the tomato sauce. Then layer the remaining ingredients as follows:

one third of the eggplant slices
one third of the remaining sauce
half the mozzarella slices
one third of the eggplant slices
one third of the sauce
half the grated Parmesan cheese
the remaining eggplant
the remaining sauce
the remaining mozzarella
the remaining Parmesan

Top with the chopped fresh parsley.

Bake 40 minutes at 400 degrees, remove from the oven, and allow to sit for at least 15 minutes before serving.

Makes 6 to 8 servings.

Nutritional information per serving (roughly): 600 calories, 40 grams total fat (13 grams saturated fat, 22 grams monounsaturated fat) (Note: For a low-fat variation, use only ¹⁄₃ cup of olive oil, ¹⁄₂ pound of mozzarella cheese, and ¹⁄₂ cup of Parmesan cheese.)

❧ QUESTIONS AND ANSWERS

❧ *What cuts of meat are the lowest in fat?*

In general, look for cuts of meat with the words "round" or "loin," such as ground round, pork loin, beef tenderloin, and so on. For beef, choose extra-lean ground beef (95 percent lean), eye of round, top round steak and roast, sirloin, or beef tenderloin. Bacon is much higher in fat than lean ham or Canadian bacon. A broiled pork chop has far less fat than pork ribs. The lowest-fat cuts of pork are pork tenderloin, top loin roast, top loin chop, center loin chop, sirloin roast, loin rib chop, and shoulderblade steak. White meat chicken and turkey are leaner than dark meat. Lamb and veal are naturally lower in fat than beef if you can find them, afford them, and want to eat them.

See the following chart for a comparison of fat content in different types of meat products. All figures are for cooked meat, generally broiled or roasted, in 3.5-ounce portions. Other portion sizes used are 3 ounces for fish, 8 ounces for milk, and 1 ounce for cheese.

	Saturated Fat Grams	*Total Fat Grams*
Eggs (1 large)	1.60	5.30
Ground beef	8.10	20.70
Ground beef, extra lean	6.40	16.30
Halibut	.40	2.50

	Saturated Fat Grams	Total Fat Grams
Ham, extra lean	1.40	4.30
Lamb, leg of, lean	3.30	9.40
Lambchop, lean	3.70	9.80
Pork tenderloin, lean	1.70	4.80
Poultry, dark meat with skin	4.40	15.80
Poultry, dark meat without skin	2.70	9.70
Poultry, light meat with skin	3.00	10.80
Poultry, light meat without skin	1.30	4.50
Salmon	2.10	10.50
Shrimp	.20	.90

✺ What is the fat content of different cheeses?

We have categorized cheeses by the amount of fat that they contain. Nonfat cheeses (as well as other nonfat dairy products) contain no fat. Low-fat cheeses and dairy products contain 3 grams of fat or less per serving. Lower-fat cheeses are those cheeses that have about 5 grams of fat or less per serving. Higher-fat cheeses contain more than 5 grams of fat per serving. The following table should help to decipher the fat content of some commonly used cheeses.

Cheese per 1-ounce Serving	Fat Grams	Saturated Fat Grams
Blue cheese	8.1	5.3
Brie	7.8	4.9
Camembert	6.9	4.3
Cheddar	9.4	6.0
Cheddar, low fat	2.0	1.2
Colby	8.7	5.5
Cottage cheese, 1% fat (1 cup)	2.3	1.5
Edam	7.9	5.0
Feta	6.0	5.4
Gruyère	9.2	5.4
Mozzarella, part skim	4.5	2.9
Mozzarella, whole milk	6.0	3.7
Parmesan, grated (1 tablespoon)	1.5	1.0
Provolone	7.5	4.8
Ricotta, part skim (½ cup)	9.8	6.1
Ricotta, whole milk (½ cup)	16.1	10.3
Romano, grated (1 tablespoon)	1.5	1.0
Swiss	7.8	4.5

❧ *What are the best ways to cook meat to reduce fat content?*

When preparing ground meat, cook, drain, and then rinse in a colander to remove excess fat. Broil or grill meat rather than frying. Use just a little olive oil or even nonfat cooking spray to keep leaner cuts from sticking to broilers and baking pans. When baking meat, use a rack so the fat drains into the bottom of the baking pan.

❧ *I feel deprived if my meal doesn't include meat. Am I doomed to high blood cholesterol levels?*

Not at all. Refer back to our section on phasing out meat main-course mentality. Even if it takes awhile, you can probably find recipes you enjoy that don't include meat. Even if you do choose to eat meat more often than is recommended in the Mediterranean Diet Pyramid, you don't have to eat it in large amounts. Stick to lean cuts of meat and reduce portion sizes. Learn to use meat in recipes instead of on its own (see recipes starting on page 225) and you'll find that what you thought was a single serving can easily serve four people. Even if you like to eat meat (as did the people eating a traditional Mediterranean diet), why not expand your culinary horizons to include an equal appreciation of the vast variety of plant foods available to you?

If you feel deprived, you won't enjoy your food, and that is certainly not in the Mediterranean spirit. Eating should be a pleasurable and fulfilling as well as filling experience. If that means including meat four or five times a week for now, that will be the plan that works for you. As long as your fat intake and saturated fat intake remain at a sensible level (no more than 30 percent of your average daily calories from fat, no more than 10 percent from saturated fat), you should be able to maintain a healthy heart.

If, however, you already suffer from high blood cholesterol and are at risk for heart disease, you may need to learn to overcome your feelings of deprivation and trim your meat intake down to the levels suggested in the Mediterranean Diet Pyramid, or even lower. Talk to your doctor about what you should be eating and how much meat makes sense for you.

🕉 *What about other, less common types of meat? How do they fit into the Mediterranean Way of eating?*

Although we didn't include game meat in our Mediterranean Diet Pyramid, since it isn't commonly consumed in this country on a regular basis, it was consumed in the traditional Mediterranean diet. If you can find it, or if you choose to go out and hunt it, fit game meats into the Mediterranean Diet Pyramid as if they were red meat, in terms of frequency of consumption and portion size. A few additional considerations:

- Water buffalo is very low in fat, with only 1.8 total grams of fat in a 3.5-ounce roasted portion, only .6 grams being saturated fat. This is a lean meat.
- Deer is also relatively low in fat, with only 3.2 grams of total fat and 1.3 grams of saturated fat in 3.5 ounces roasted meat.
- Eel is high in fat, with 12.7 grams of total fat and 2.6 grams of saturated fat in a 3-ounce portion cooked over dry heat.

- Elk is a lean meat, with 1.9 total grams of fat and only .7 grams of saturated fat in a 3.5-ounce serving of roasted meat.
- Goat is also a lean meat, with 3.0 grams of total fat and .9 grams of saturated fat in a 3.5-ounce portion of roasted meat.

❧ Are free-range chickens more heart-healthy?

Not necessarily. Free-range chickens probably aren't any different in their fat, protein, vitamin, and mineral content. However, some people believe they taste better. Also, some free-range chickens are raised on food without antibiotics, growth hormones, and other additives, and this is preferable to some. On the other hand, free-range chickens tend to be more expensive.

❧ Should I buy shrimp from the guy in the van selling it on the street corner?

We wouldn't. It could be that the shrimp—or lobster or crab legs or whatever is being offered—is just fine. On the other hand, seafood spoils quickly, meaning that if it isn't properly refrigerated, bacteria growth can reach dangerous levels. Buy fish from a dependable source.

❧ Which fish should go in which recipes?

Lower-fat fish—the kind that is lighter in color, like orange roughy and sole—is best for baking and cooking in the microwave. Fattier fish, such as salmon, tuna, and mackerel (the types with higher fat content but also higher omega-3 fat content) are ideal for grilling and broiling.

❧ *How do I know if fish is fresh?*

Fresh fish smells pleasantly like the sea with flesh that is firm, translucent, moist, and without brown spots. Mollusks like clams and mussels should be alive when purchased with undamaged, slightly open shells that close when tapped. Scallops should be moist and plump, and shrimp will smell "shrimpy" but not strongly. If any fish smells unpleasant, don't buy it.

Frozen fish should be frozen completely solid and without crystals or dry, discolored spots. It should have only a slight odor and be well wrapped.

Even if the fish you buy is fresh when you buy it, it won't stay that way for long. Eat fish and seafood the day you buy it or the next day. If you won't eat it that soon, freeze it, but fish that has already been frozen will deteriorate in quality if refrozen. Best to buy seafood the day you plan to prepare it.

8: *Embracing the Mediterranean Lifestyle*

Compare the typical day of an American man, let's say about forty years old, with that of a typical farmer of the same age living in the rural Mediterranean in 1950. Of course, we never lived in the Mediterranean region at this time, but we can make an educated guess about what life may have been like.

Both the American man and the Mediterranean man rise at about six A.M., the American man with the aid of an alarm clock that drags him from a groggy haze after a scant five hours of sleep, the Mediterranean man waking naturally with the first rays of the sun over the horizon after a satisfying eight hours of sleep.

The American man grabs a doughnut and a cup of coffee with white sugar and hydrogenated nondairy creamer at a convenience store on the way to the office. The Mediterranean man sits down to a light breakfast of whole-grain bread and coffee with hot milk.

The American man gets frustrated and angry sitting in traffic for an hour. He sees nothing but concrete, overpasses, underpasses, interchanges, and other cars. The Mediterranean man opens his front door and is already at work. He breathes deeply the fresh, cool morning air and pauses momentarily to watch the sun rise over the lovely green hills of his farm. The distant sea sparkles.

All day, the American man sits at a desk in front of a computer screen except for a walk into the neighboring conference room for a long meeting. He is often on the phone, on line, or immersed in writing a report. His eyes ache but none of his other muscles do much moving at all. He breaks for lunch at one o'clock with his colleagues. His order might consist of a bacon cheeseburger or a corned beef on rye, French fries, a slice of cheesecake, and a large cola, or perhaps even a martini or two. He leaves work wearily at seven P.M.

All day, the Mediterranean man works hard in the field. His entire body gets a great workout, although he doesn't think of his efforts as "exercise." They are, quite simply, what one does. He breaks midmorning for another hearty slab of whole-grain bread, and again for lunch, the biggest meal of his day: more bread wrapped around a handful of greens cooked in olive oil with a little lemon or vinegar, a piece of cheese, a glass of red wine, and a slice of melon for dessert. Back to the fields, the man works vigorously in the fresh air. The work is hard and tiring, and his muscles ache, but he sees the results of his work there before him—a newly plowed field, an acre of harvested olives, or a neatly tended vineyard.

The American man stops at the gym on his way home for a game of racquetball with a friend. He loses and it irritates him exceedingly. He drives home in a bad temper, picks up a pepperoni pizza for his family, and he, his wife, and his two children eat the pizza in silence in front of a blaring television. The television stays on long after the children have gone to bed, and he watches it late into the night.

The Mediterranean man also works until about seven P.M. Tired and hungry, he comes home to a light salad, a dish of pasta, a glass of red wine, and a bowl of citrus fruit. He eats with his family. They talk. Perhaps the family from the neighboring farm joins them for the light meal. They exchange stories, the news of the village, farming or cooking tips. When the sun is fully set, everyone goes off to bed.

Which lifestyle sounds healthier? Of course, we've certainly oversimplified and, admittedly, romanticized the Mediterranean lifestyle in our description. Life was certainly hard for the working classes in the Mediterranean region. Money was often tight for farmers and laborers. A natural disaster or a physical injury could destroy a crop and a family's income for the year. Work must surely have been stressful more often than not. Children got sick. People didn't always agree. Sometimes there wasn't enough food to satisfy everyone.

But we compare the two—the American man and the Mediterranean man—to make a point: In the traditional Mediterranean, life was, most certainly, three things: technologically simple, physically rigorous, and in touch with the natural world.

Not incidentally, although we used a man for our example, women's lives in the traditional Mediterranean were similarly physically active—cooking by hand without appliances, washing clothes without machines, washing dishes without machines, sweeping and dusting and scrubbing the home without machines or chemical cleaners, sewing clothes, gardening, going into town to shop, taking care of the children. And American women, of course, lead lives much like American men.

Could the Mediterranean lifestyle be a factor in the superior coronary health and longevity of the traditional Mediterranean people? Research says probably, and why wouldn't it? Study after study has demonstrated that exercise, in whatever form, lowers the risk and also the severity of many chronic diseases, from heart disease to depression.

Chronic stress—which may be the result of a complicated lifestyle as well as a lifestyle largely removed from the natural world—has been linked to any number of health problems. While people in the traditional Mediterranean undoubtedly experienced stress—in other words, that physical fight-or-flight response to certain stimuli our bodies undergo, preparing us to deal with crisis— chronic stress over a period of months, even years, was probably far less prevalent than it is today in our overextended and hectic world.

The irony of life in the traditional Mediterranean was that, on the surface, it looked a lot more stressful than contemporary American life. Not enough food, never enough meat, hard physical labor day in and day out, an existence at the mercy of the elements and luck, large families in small living spaces, none of the modern conveniences of living.

Yet, for all our conveniences—cars, central heating, cable television, computers, overhead lights, fax machines, programmable coffee makers, credit cards, electric razors, clock radios, cellular phones, burglar alarms, riding mowers—we've sacrificed a life close to the earth, full of movement and strength-building activity, in physical contact with our friends and even strangers. We've lost much of the old sense of community, of knowing and depending on our neighbors, of doing a job and seeing the result right there in front of us, of earning the money and using it to buy what we need, of building our own homes, growing our own foods, even of moving our own bodies.

What price have we paid for modern life? And can we ever reclaim some of the simpler aspects of life so taken for granted by people living the traditional Mediterranean culture? Can we regain a sense of community, relearn how to live simply, and recapture an active lifestyle without sacrificing the jobs we love, the cars we need, the beautiful houses with our names on the mortgages, the conveniences that have become so necessary to get along in contemporary society?

Of course we can. We can have it all! It just takes a little planning, and a few priority adjustments. But first, let's look at the evidence, so we can be sure that moving toward a more Mediterranean-inspired lifestyle is really worth the effort.

� TO MOVE IS TO LIVE

Physical activity was par for the course in the rural Mediterranean. People had to be active and endure often grueling physical labor just to make a living and get food on the table. We, on the other hand, often have to make time for exercise. It has to be something we "pencil in" to our busy schedules, and it is, all too frequently, the first thing to be crossed off the list when those schedules get too tight. You have to finish that report, or get to the grocery store, or drive the kids to soccer practice, or serve on that committee. The half-hour run through the park you had planned can wait . . . can't it?

Maybe not, if you want to stay healthy enough to write that report or pick up that gallon of milk. Studies on both men and women make compelling arguments that exercise is literally a matter of life and death.

A study published in a 1999 issue of the *New England Journal of Medicine* revealed that women who walk briskly for at least three hours each week or who exercise more vigorously—jogging or aerobic dance—for ninety minutes per week reduce their heart attack risk by 30 to

40 percent, and women who walk for five or more hours per week cut their heart attack risk in half.

Even shorter periods of exercise can have a positive effect on heart health. Research out of Loughborough University in Leicestershire, England, demonstrated that shorter exercise sessions—ten minutes three times per day rather than 30 minutes all at once—can indeed lower heart attack risk in young, healthy men by lowering triglyceride levels after meals.

Exercise can do more than cut your heart attack risk. Research out of the University of Illinois suggests that older people who begin a program of aerobic exercise such as walking can maintain their mental "fitness" better than older people who remain sedentary. The study examined sedentary adults between sixty and seventy-five years old and asked them to begin either walking or a stretching and toning program. After six months, mental reactions in the walking group (who worked up to forty-five-minute walks at about 3.8 miles per hour three times per week) were up to 25 percent quicker than mental reactions in the stretching and toning group.

A two-year study conducted at the Cooper Institute for Aerobics Research in Dallas, Texas, studied a similar subject: the effect of more total aerobic activity each day accomplished piecemeal throughout the day, rather than in one chunk of structured exercise time. They found that many of the participants not only lowered their blood cholesterol levels but also lost excess weight.

Why is exercise so good for our bodies? An easier question may be, why is a lack of physical activity so bad for our bodies? It is a scientifically noted reality that people who live sedentary lives are more prone to a variety of chronic diseases such as heart disease, stroke, colon cancer, diabetes, and osteoporosis. Inactive people tend to suffer more often from obesity. They don't seem to live as long. On a less dramatic scale, physically active people tend to have fewer colds, better sleep, and a more positive attitude than the sedentary. Isn't that reason enough to get up and get moving?

Exercise benefits the entire body in a multitude of ways. Physical activity lowers blood cholesterol levels, and more specifically, lowers LDL ("bad") cholesterol levels. One study of men and postmenopausal women with elevated LDL cholesterol levels (a risk factor for heart disease) on either no treatment, an exercise plan, or the National Cholesterol Education Program Step 2 diet, showed the exercisers alone to be successful in lowering their levels of LDL cholesterol.

Exercise helps prevent high blood pressure and also lowers already high blood pressure levels. Physical activity strengthens the heart muscle, helping it to work more efficiently. It also appears to lower the levels of certain immune system chemicals in the blood that promote atherosclerosis, and increase levels of certain chemicals that prevent atherosclerosis.

Exercise improves your body's ability to metabolize carbohydrates, increasing sensitivity to insulin and lowering the risk of developing adult-onset diabetes, which some believe is actually a disease of inactivity. Exercise also helps to move waste through your digestive system more quickly, which may be the mechanism whereby it lowers colon cancer risk—if toxins and carcinogens are in your digestive tract for less time, they have less chance of being absorbed by the body. Weight-bearing exercise strengthens bones, reducing the risk of developing osteoporosis.

Perhaps most compelling is the effect of physical activity on longevity. One British study showed that moderate exercise appeared to reduce the risk of death in older men. The death risk of moderately active men was half that of sedentary men, and deaths from all causes were highest among sedentary men.

Another study from the Cooper Institute for Aerobics Research in Dallas shows that among people with the same illness, those who exercise live longer. A study of physical activity and mortality in postmenopausal women concluded that any kind of exercise seems to lower the risk of death in postmenopausal women. The study included postmenopausal subjects and found that the more women exercised, the lower their risk of death during the study's follow-up period. Even women who exercised only once a week experienced what the study called a "significant drop in mortality," but the women who enjoyed the lowest risk of death were those who exercised at least four times per week or who regularly exercised vigorously.

Even if exercise didn't add years to your life (which it apparently does), it certainly adds life to your years, as they say. Exercise is increasingly prescribed by physicians as a treatment for chronic diseases, from cancer to high blood pressure, diabetes to arthritis. Exercise can make the elderly stronger and more independent.

❧ HERCULES WAS GREEK

As important as aerobic exercise is for your health, strength training is equally important. You probably couldn't find someone in the traditional Mediterranean lifting weights, and you don't have to, either. But you can work more weight-bearing activity into your day.

In the Mediterranean, weight-bearing activities were a part of life on a farm: lifting, hauling, pulling, loading, pushing, chopping, digging. Americans don't do much of these activities anymore unless by choice, or unless they choose farming or some form of manual labor as a profession. Yet, strength training can easily become a part of modern American life, even without having to purchase an expensive set of freeweights.

Strength training requires less endurance but more short-term intense effort. Weight-bearing exercises not only build muscle, they also build bone. Studies indicate that older people who begin a strength-training program show improved muscle tone and function, improved bone density, and greater strength.

Stronger muscles do more than look better. They work better. We don't mean huge, bulky, incapacitating muscles (which are difficult to achieve, anyway, especially for women, who don't typically have the necessary testosterone). We mean fit, fully nourished, active muscles. Larger muscle cells more accustomed to moving can process oxygen better, taking some of the load off the hard-working heart muscle, which doesn't have to "push" so hard to supply those muscles with nutrients. Strong muscles surrounding arthritic joints help to take the pressure off joints. Muscle strength can also make small differences all day long—that grocery bag isn't such a load, those sacks of lawn trash are trifles, those twin toddlers aren't so heavy after all, even when they jump on you simultaneously.

Work weight-bearing activity into your daily life by doing more things for yourself: carrying grocery bags, packages, small children; shoveling snow, raking leaves, digging in the garden; even walking up and down stairs lifts the body weight. Many people enjoy yoga, which employs weight bearing by lifting and manipulating the weight of the body in a controlled manner.

Whatever method you choose, don't forget that aerobic

activity and weight-bearing activity go hand in hand, working together to improve your health.

� NO TIME TO LOSE

But you've heard this story. You know exercise is good for you. Yet, you still have trouble fitting it into your schedule. We live in a nation of convenience. Where else would you find convenience stores on every other corner? These stores do well because Americans truly believe they don't have enough time to do it all.

Do you think you don't have time to exercise? Do you think you don't have the energy? The important thing to remember is that regular exercise will give you more energy, which will make you feel as if you have more time. Some other tips for fitting exercise into your day are as follows:

- Remember that exercise in bits and pieces throughout the day is just as effective as exercise all in one session, as long as the total time and exertion is the same.
- Climb up and down the stairs in your home or office as often as possible. Forget elevators.
- Park in the most distant parking space from your destination. Think of the time you'll save circling the parking lot looking for the choicest space! And your car will be easier to find.
- Save gas, save the environment, and save your muscle tone—walk everywhere possible! While some cities and environments are less conducive to pedestrians than others, you may find plenty of opportunities for walking you hadn't consid-

ered. Some people even drive to their mailboxes, or to the next-door neighbor's house. That need not be you.

- If you take the bus or subway to and from work, get off a stop or two earlier and walk the rest of the way. Wear your athletic shoes and carry your work shoes.

- If you work at a computer all day, make it a habit to get up every fifteen minutes and stretch. A brisk three-minute walk around the office or outside every hour or two is even better.

- Put your cooking machines away behind closed cupboard doors. Only get them out when you really need them. You can knead bread dough, whip up cake batter, or beat eggs by hand.

- If your attempts to exercise always fail because you've planned to get up earlier and exercise in the morning, change your plan. Some people have a higher energy level later in the day. A brisk walk right after work each day might suit you better, or maybe an evening run is more your speed (if so, wear reflective gear—not a necessity in the Mediterranean but an important safety precaution in our busy cities).

- Play with the kids (or the dog). Don't let the shorter members of your household play in the backyard or the park alone. Engage them in a game of tag, keep-away, Frisbee, or whatever game is "cool" in school this week. Not only will you get some great exercise, but you'll be engaging in family time, an essential part of the traditional Mediterranean lifestyle.

- Exercise with your partner or friend. If you aren't in the mood, your buddy can talk you back into the mood, and vice versa. Jog together, play tennis, ride bicycles, rollerblade, swim, even mall-walk. Exercise is more fun when you've got someone to talk to, and once again, such a social endeavor is certainly in the Mediterranean spirit.

- Don't hire the neighborhood kids to do your lawn chores. Do them yourself. Rake the leaves, weed the garden, mow, shovel snow. You'll get exercise and a sense of accomplishment when you see the results. You'll also save the money you would have paid to have the service performed for you.

- Instead of spending your weekend night out at a movie, go dancing, ice skating, or roller-skating.

- Getting together with friends? Why not go canoeing or cross-country skiing? Hit the courts for a friendly game of basketball, or the green for a game of golf (without the golf carts, of course!).

- Turn off the TV! The more active alternative activities are staggering in number and variety. Go for a walk. Clean your closet. Visit the zoo or the museum. Organize your pantry alphabetically. Scrub the bathtub. Dance to your favorite music. Jump rope. Bring in a load of firewood. Chop more firewood! Or, if you absolutely must have the television on, pop in an exercise video and get off that couch!

- If you like your exercise in a more spiritual form, take a yoga, tai chi, or martial arts class. Not Mediterranean, but exercise is exercise!

❦ A MEDITERRANEAN-INSPIRED EXERCISE PLAN

The American College of Sports Medicine recently recommended that everyone, no matter their age, shape, or fitness level, should exercise for at least thirty minutes per day on most days of the week. For weight loss, the ACSM recommends forty-five to sixty minutes of aerobic activity each day. Strength training is important, too.

That may sound like a lot, but if you follow our Mediterranean-Inspired Three-Day Exercise Plan, you'll find that the recommendation is actually fairly easy to accomplish. And fun too! The beauty of this plan is its simplicity. You don't need equipment, special instruction, or even any special skills. You just need to know how to walk.

The following plan is just a guide. You can follow it exactly or you can tailor it to your own needs. You can increase or decrease the length or intensity of any of the activities. You can mix and match activities. You can do the plan for three days and take a day off, or do some version of the plan every day. (This plan isn't so strenuous as to require a day off. It can be performed every day.)

The intensity at which you exercise is dependent on your fitness level. You should feel like you are working hard, but not so hard that you can't carry on a conversation. Sweat, but don't knock yourself out. Don't think a leisurely stroll around the block will do the trick either, however. Remember—move it or lose it!

Day One

- Do five minutes of gentle stretching and fifty jumping jacks before breakfast (or start with five jumping jacks and work your way up to fifty). Good morning!
- For your midmorning coffee break, take a brisk ten-minute walk (in the fresh air, if possible).
- Take a fifteen-minute walk during lunch.
- Before dinner, either at your job or elsewhere, find a flight of stairs and go up and down a few times.
- End your day with as many sit-ups and push-ups

as you can do with some effort but without pain (increase by a few repetitions every week or two), and finally, some gentle stretching. If you have kids, they'll probably be happy to join you on the floor, and you can set a great example!

Day Two

- Begin your day with gentle stretching, then march in place briskly for five minutes.
- Take the bus to work and get off one stop early. Walk the rest of the way (ten minutes).
- Move more, eat less. Pack a light lunch and take a fifteen-minute walk.
- For your afternoon coffee break, do some stair climbing.
- Before dinner, go on a bike ride with a friend (or play a game of tennis, golf, or do some in-line skating).

Day Three

- Begin your day with gentle stretching, then put on some wake-up music and dance for five minutes.
- Rally your coworkers and take a brisk, twenty-minute lunchtime walk.
- For your afternoon coffee break, jog in place for two minutes, do ten jumping jacks, then try twenty push-ups against a wall. You won't need the coffee!
- After a light supper, enlist your partner, children, or your dog for a brisk, fifteen-minute (or more) evening walk.
- Before bed, grab two cans of food (or one- to two-pound weights, if you have them), hold one in each hand, and see how long you can keep your arms extended. Then try your sit-ups with

the cans of food held against your chest, for extra weight.

❧ STRESS AND THE BODY

We don't want to give the impression that people living in the Mediterranean and eating a traditional Mediterranean diet didn't experience stress. Contemporary America is plagued by a different kind of stress, however—an insidious, chronic stress that often goes unrecognized. People who have all their basic needs met—food, clothing, shelter, warmth—fall prey to stresses from other sources. Financial difficulties, difficulties with relationships, demanding careers or jobs, parenting, or any number of other stresses can become sources of long-term, chronic stress.

Exercise can help your body deal with stress more efficiently. Even if you exercise daily, however, you probably are still under plenty of stress. What is stress, exactly? Stress is a reaction in the body, sometimes called the fight-or-flight reaction, that prepares the body to handle extreme circumstances. Stress can be a good thing, and a survival mechanism. If we are confronted with danger, our body prepares us to react quickly to preserve our lives and the lives of those we protect.

When we sense danger (whether an approaching tiger or an approaching exam or an approaching speech), our bodies do certain things, all triggered by the release of two stress hormones, adrenaline and corticotrophin-releasing hormone. These hormones induce certain physical changes in the body:

- Blood platelets clump together, in preparation for a potential wound (to stop any bleeding).

- The immune system activates in readiness for trauma.
- Blood and blood sugar rush to the extremities and the muscles to prepare them for action.
- Muscles contract in readiness.
- Heart rate and breathing rate speed up and blood pressure rises.

After the danger has passed, a steroid hormone called cortisol signals the body to return to its normal state. The problem is that in modern life, some people are under so much stress that the body fails to return to its normal state. In others, cortisol, for whatever reason, doesn't signal the body as it should. The stressed or fight-or-flight state is not intended to be a permanent or long-term state. The immune system reverses its elevated function and becomes depressed, leaving the stressed person vulnerable. The clumping action of blood platelets over the long term can increase the risk of heart attacks. Too much cortisol in the body can depress immune function, trigger bone loss, and increase insulin production. One study on aging animals and humans links chronically high levels of stress hormones to memory loss.

The entire chemical process that takes place in a body under stress can go awry in many ways, but the upshot is that gearing our lifestyles to reduce stress is both healthier for our bodies and for our overextended minds. It is also quintessentially Mediterranean.

ℬ PEOPLE WHO NEED ...

In traditional Mediterranean culture, people had many mechanisms for dealing with stress. Family bonds were often strong and of utmost priority. Friends and neigh-

bors supported each other, helped each other when someone was in need, and spent time together.

People were also closer to the natural world than many
of us are today. They worked the land, they spent time
outdoors, and they weren't isolated most of the time from
the natural world by cars, insulated and sealed homes,
shopping malls, and hermetically sealed office buildings.

Whether exposure to nature has an effect on stress levels
may be a matter of debate. Research on the subject is slim,
but anecdotal evidence supports the theory. A more studied
area concerns strong social ties as a weapon against stress.
Strong friendships and a social network of support may
strengthen the immune system, slow the aging process,
reduce disease risk, even increase longevity.

A 1989 Stanford University study demonstrated that
women with metastatic breast cancer who were involved
in support groups lived an average of eighteen months
longer than those who were not in a support group, and
other research has demonstrated highly active natural
killer cells in cancer patients who say they feel emotion-
ally supported. Social support, it is theorized, increases
white blood cell activity by decreasing stress.

Another investigation published in a 1997 issue of the
Journal of the American Medical Association linked a
lack of diverse social contacts to an increased risk of
developing colds—even more of an increased risk than
for smokers, people with low vitamin C intakes, or people with elevated stress hormones!

❦ LOW-STRESS LIVING

But how do we engage in more low-stress living?
Moving to southern Italy or to a Greek island and living
off the land with our best friends may sound nice, but it

isn't very practical for most. Yet, we can capture the spirit of such a life even as we continue living in our fast-paced society. Here are some tips:

- **Cherish your friends.** Nurture and expand your social contacts. If you sometimes feel isolated and unable to meet people, ask family members or acquaintances for ideas. Support groups, community groups, religious organizations, and universities or community colleges often have groups open to interested members of the community.

- **Try meditation.** Many techniques can be effective for relieving stress. We like visualization. Spend five or ten minutes each morning and each evening in solitude, eyes closed. Envision wandering the Grecian coastline, relaxing in a café in southern France, strolling through a museum in Florence, basking in the sun on a beach in southern Spain. A mini-vacation every day can recharge you and help your body to remember how relaxation feels.

- **Spend a little time outside every day.** Let the sun warm your skin (but wear a sunscreen!). Feel the breeze. Breathe the fresh air. If you live in a place where fresh air is at a premium, make it a point to drive out of the city at least every few weeks so you can recall what the natural world looks like! In the meantime, plant a patio or windowsill garden with a few flowers or fresh herbs. Even in the winter months, you can enjoy, even cherish, the outdoors. Many of us who live in wintry climates know well the sense of calm and exhilaration of walking through new-fallen snow (stay safe, of course, and don't walk in blizzards or on icy pavement).

- **Put things in perspective.** So your toddler spilled a gallon of milk on the floor, your report blew out the window of your car, your son wants to join a heavy-metal rock band, and your computer crashed. These things may be inconvenient, irritating, even life changing, but they needn't throw you off course to such an extent that you get sick. Remember the Serenity Prayer about accepting what you can't change, changing what you can, and being wise enough to know the difference? The words are of Irish, not Mediterranean, origin, but their wisdom is universal.

- **Exercise every day.** The world will seem like a much nicer place. Whenever possible, forego the convenient machine and do things by hand.

- **Speak your mind—within reason.** Telling people how you feel and what you think may help to relieve stress if you can air your anxieties and get problems out into the open. On the other hand, speaking in anger may result in saying things you don't mean, which can cause more stress in the future. Your best bet may be to talk out your anxieties and worries with an unbiased or sympathetic third party—family members, friends, your partner, or a counselor.

- **Write about it.** A 1999 study of people with asthma or rheumatoid arthritis revealed better health among those who kept a journal to express their feelings about stressful events in their lives. Writing how you feel can be a great outlet for stress, and it doesn't hurt anyone's feelings!

- **Embrace life.** Live in the here and now and treasure every moment rather than letting your days slip away unlived. Savor your food, stop and enjoy a beautiful view, take time out for a

walk in the fresh air, take a hot bath, really listen
to your loved ones, and try to experience everything you do rather than living on "automatic
pilot."

- **Offer support, and ask for it.** Take advantage
of your friends and family in the best way, by
being there for them and letting them be there
for you. A long-term HIV-infected "nonprogres-
sor" (someone who has the HIV virus but has
remained healthy without developing full-blown
AIDS) named Stephen Foster described what
other long-term HIV survivors have in common: "This is a generalization, but people who
are long-term survivors seem to be more concerned about living than dying. Instead of
depending solely on pharmaceuticals, they
reach out to as many types of support as are
available to them. They do not isolate themselves, and they are willing to ask for support
and give it to others."

- **Don't smoke and don't drink excessively.** One
or two glasses of red wine per day is more than
enough alcohol for some people.

- **Make relaxation a priority.** Schedule in five or
ten minutes each day to relax profoundly, undis-
turbed. Consider it an investment toward produc-
tivity and efficient functioning.

- **Rechannel your anger.** Anger can elevate cholesterol levels, raise blood pressure, and has been
linked to depression. One of the best ways to
control anger is to raise your exercise level and to
identify things that trigger your anger and avoid
them. When something bothers you, let people
know instead of repressing your feelings. If your
anger is out of control, seek counseling. A pro-

fessional counselor can help you learn to deal
with your anger.
- **Don't forget to follow the Mediterranean Diet
Pyramid.**

❧ QUESTIONS AND ANSWERS

❧ *How much longer do people live who exercise
regularly?*

About two to three years, which may not sound like
much, but is slightly longer than the amount of time average longevity would increase if all cancer was completely eliminated tomorrow.

❧ *Are certain activities more effective for certain health
problems like heart disease or arthritis?*

Most moderate exercise is beneficial for most health
problems, but some conditions necessitate an adjustment
in an exercise plan. For example, arthritis can make exercise painful, so good ways to strengthen the heart and the
muscles with minimal stress to joints include low-impact
exercise like swimming and walking; stretching and toning exercise like yoga; and strength training.

Strength training is important for people suffering
from osteoporosis. Studies show weight-bearing exercise
may actually stop or reverse bone density loss.

Aerobic exercise appears to be most beneficial for diabetes, and moderate aerobic exercise works best for high
blood pressure. Depression seems to respond to both aerobic exercise, especially in a social or group setting, and
weight training.

✤ *Do people need more or less exercise as they age?*

More. Unfortunately, people tend to get less and less the older they become. As we age, our muscle strength and flexibility decrease, our endurance decreases, and hormonal changes can speed up certain changes such as loss of bone density. Exercise can halt or counteract many of these changes, making old age largely a matter of numbers, not of limitations.

✤ *Exercise is so boring! I can't keep it up for more than a couple of weeks.*

Exercise needn't be boring, and is most often considered boring by those who have a relatively narrow view of what exercise is. Simply doing more for yourself rather than relying on automation can raise your activity level. Walk more, and walk faster. Spend your spare time moving—playing games, bicycling, swimming, or again, walking. You don't need to join a fitness club or buy any equipment to enjoy a more active lifestyle. See the tips on page 247 for fitting more exercise into your life.

✤ *I live in an area where air pollution is a problem. Should I still exercise outdoors?*

Exercising in air pollution can actually be detrimental to your health, increasing your risk of heart disease, suppressing your immune system, and increasing your chances of developing respiratory problems. Runners take in ten times the air per minute as people standing still, and if that air is polluted, those pollutants enter your body ten times faster. If you have allergies or asthma, you are at an even greater risk of developing health problems from exercising in a polluted environment.

As nice as outdoor exercise is, if you live in a polluted environment, your best bet probably is to exercise indoors, whether that means finding a walking track at a local gym, joining a fitness center, or walking the local mall with your buddies. Whenever possible, take a day trip or a vacation to a nonpolluted area and take advantage of the fresh air by staying as active as possible.

In general, air pollution is at its worst during the hottest part of the day, so exercising in the early morning or evening will expose you to slightly cleaner air. If you hear on the news that pollution levels are high on a given day, stay inside. Don't walk or run near high-traffic areas, if possible. May to September is smog season, so summer may be the best time to exercise inside if you live in a big city.

✺ Is exercise important for children?

Yes! Obesity and even high cholesterol are increasing problems for American kids today. Too much television and too many video games? Too much junk food? Whatever the reason, the results are real. Encourage kids to get outside and stay active. Stock the cupboards and refrigerator with healthy snacks like fresh fruits, vegetables, and whole-grain bread and crackers. Low-fat cheese, low-fat milk, and low-fat yogurt are good snacks, too. The Mediterranean Diet Pyramid is also meant for children over the age of two. Perhaps most important, set a good example for your kids. If they see you eating healthy foods and staying active, they will want to do the same (even if they won't admit it!).

♋ *My job is very stressful. Should I quit?*

All jobs are stressful some of the time. If your job is a source of extreme stress in your life, however, you may want to consider what about your job is causing you so much displeasure. Is it the working environment? The people? Are your skills underutilized or have you neglected to follow your dream?

We strongly support finding a life's work that engages and excites you. This can be a source of great pleasure and satisfaction. However, you may be able to fulfill this need with a hobby, a small business on the side, or as another sort of part-time venture while keeping the job that provides you with security. If you are in a position to quit and follow your dream without risking the health or livelihood of people who depend on you, then why not go for it? It never hurts to have a sensible backup plan just in case. You should also have a realistic, researched, and detailed plan of action. However, you may be one of those who can someday say, "I lived my dream!"

♋ *The Mediterranean lifestyle sounds perfect for me. Should I move there?*

Ah, the dream of many. Keep in mind that the Mediterranean has changed a lot since the days when Ancel Keys was researching the traditional Mediterranean diet. Many of our modern conveniences have entered the region and transformed it. There are still plenty of rustic and rural pockets left, however, and lots of really great food.

You may be able to satisfy much of your Mediterranean longing by reading. Travel accounts abound, and tourist guides for the area are also in plentiful supply in bookstores. Browse the Internet for Mediterranean information, recipes, and traveling tips.

If you have the means, you might also consider vacationing in the Mediterranean. Try the food, the climate, and the lifestyle out for yourself. Consider a hiking tour or other active endeavor, and don't forget the local cuisine. Just remember to eat like the people in the Mediterranean eat, not like the tourists eat. You'll save yourself a twenty-pound weight gain.

If you do visit, write us a letter and tell us how you liked it. We wish we were there right now!

❧ *Is the Mediterranean diet and lifestyle really something practical to live with every day in America?*

The Mediterranean Diet Pyramid, an active lifestyle, more contact with the natural world, strong social ties, a sense of community, and diligent practice of stress-management techniques? Why, this is modern living at its finest. Welcome to the twenty-first century!

Appendix

🍃 ONE WEEK OF MEALS IN THE MEDITERRANEAN SPIRIT

You've got the will. Now we'll give you the way. To help launch your new mode of eating in the true spirit of the traditional Mediterranean diet, we've provided a week's worth of meals. This is by no means a strict diet you must follow, but simply a menu plan to provide inspiration and, if you prefer it, a little structured guidance.

Feel free to substitute similar foods for each item, to add additional fruits, veggies, and whole grains if you are still hungry, or to adjust portion sizes according to need. Everyone is an individual with differing dietary needs. The point is to eat a variety of healthy foods corresponding to the Mediterranean Diet Pyramid, and to enjoy every bite.

This menu will provide you with a well-balanced eating plan. While the menu is not designed for weight loss or gain, you might find you have so much energy and feel so good about yourself while eating it that you inch closer to the weight that is healthiest for you. We did not include beverages here, such as alcohol or coffee, because these are optional items in the Mediterranean diet plan. Including such foods in your diet is an individual decision, and should be based on your overall health status. Green tea has been given a lot of attention lately as a promoter of good health, which can also be included if you wish. Many of the recipes listed here can be found in the previous chapters.

Three important things to remember when planning your Mediterranean-inspired meals:

- Enjoy your food! Savor the texture, flavor, and color of your food. This is good eating beyond nutrition. It is a feast for the senses. The more you enjoy your food, the more Mediterranean in character your meals will be.
- Don't forget to drink lots of water! Aim for six to eight 8-ounce glasses of good-quality water each day.
- Exercise, Rest, and Relax! These three important lifestyle components can greatly affect eating habits, and are shown outside of the Mediterranean Diet Pyramid. Get outdoors and move in any way that you can, and value the importance of rest and relaxation for overall health.

✤ MONDAY

Breakfast
- 1 to 2 cups whole-grain cereal topped with a handful of dried fruit and ½ ounce dried or roasted nuts
- 1 cup low-fat or nonfat milk

Lunch
- 2 slices whole-grain bread with 1 ounce part-skim mozzarella cheese, 3 (or more) large leaves

of Romaine lettuce, 2 thick slices ripe tomato, a dash of olive oil, and a sprinkling of salt and pepper
- 1 cup vegetable soup
- 1 fresh pear

Snack
- 12 whole almonds

Dinner
- Moroccan Vegetable Stew (recipe on page 187)
- Couscous
- Green salad with shredded carrots, drizzled with Olive Oil Vinaigrette (recipe on page 84)
- Fresh berries with ½ cup of plain nonfat yogurt

❀ TUESDAY

Breakfast
- Banana bread made with olive or canola oil and whole-grain flour (1 to 2 slices, depending on size of loaf)
- ½ ounce nuts or seeds (which may also be mixed into the banana bread)
- 1 fresh orange
- 1 cup warm or steamed nonfat milk with a touch of vanilla extract mixed in, and topped with a dash of cinnamon

Lunch
- One cup pasta mixed with a bit of olive oil, topped with ½ ounce of walnut pieces, 1 tablespoon Parmesan cheese, and fresh parsley

- Green salad with Olive Oil Vinaigrette (recipe on page 84) drizzled on top
- Stuffed Peaches (recipe on page 155)

Snack
- Baby carrots with hummus dip (chickpea–sesame paste dip widely available in stores and easy to handmake with canned chickpeas and purchased sesame paste)

Dinner
- Tuscan Bean Soup (recipe on page 183)
- 1 to 2 slices whole-grain bread
- ½ to 1 ounce low-fat cheese
- Macedonia Salad (recipe on page 154)

❦ WEDNESDAY

Breakfast
- Oatmeal or other hot cereal (¾ to 1 cup dry mixed with 1 to 2 cups nonfat or low-fat milk to cook), then mixed with 1 to 2 heaping spoonfuls of pumpkin puree (or canned pumpkin), a tablespoon each of raisins, snipped dried apricots, and walnuts, and a sprinkle of brown sugar or maple syrup

Lunch
- Mashed white beans spread on whole-wheat pita bread
- Greek Salad (recipe on page 126)
- Citrus compote (recipe on page 156)

Snack
- 1 slice whole-grain toast with 1½ tablespoons peanut or almond butter

Dinner
- Basque Paella (recipe on page 188)
- Steamed broccoli tossed with olive oil, minced garlic, and a few hot pepper flakes
- ½ cup nonfat frozen yogurt topped with prune puree or berries

❦ THURSDAY

Breakfast
- Whole-grain bagel with 2 tablespoons almond or peanut butter
- 6 whole, pitted dates
- 1 cup nonfat milk

Lunch
- Mediterranean Vegetable and Walnut Salad with Olive Vinaigrette (recipe on page 189)
- ½ cup pineapple slices mixed in ½ to 1 cup of plain nonfat yogurt

Snack
- Green beans, steamed, chilled, and dipped in Olive Oil Vinaigrette (recipe on page 84)

Dinner
- Vegetable pizza topped with ½ to 1 ounce part-skim mozzarella cheese
- Stuffed Artichoke (recipe on page 127)
- Baked apple

✤ FRIDAY

Breakfast
- 1 to 2 cups whole-grain cereal, dried fruit, and ½ ounce nuts, mixed in 1 cup plain, nonfat yogurt

Lunch
- Tapenade on whole-grain sesame crackers (recipe on page 83)
- Green salad with tomatoes, ¼ ounce sliced almonds, and Olive Oil Vinaigrette (recipe on page 84)
- 1 tangerine
- 1 cup nonfat milk

Snack
- Broccoli florets dipped in a bit of plain nonfat yogurt blended with low-fat cottage cheese (half of each)

Dinner
- Seafood Risotto (recipe on page 227)
- ½ cup spinach sautéed with olive oil and minced garlic
- Grilled bananas

✤ SATURDAY

Breakfast
- Whole-grain pancakes made from scratch with olive or canola oil and nonfat milk, yogurt, or buttermilk, topped with ½ to 1 cup fresh fruit, ¾

cup nonfat yogurt, and ½ ounce nuts such as pecans, almonds, or walnuts (you can also toss the nuts into the batter)
- 1 cup nonfat milk

Lunch
- Falafel with Tomato-Cucumber Relish (recipe on page 184)
- Green salad with fresh plum tomatoes and Olive Oil Vinaigrette (recipe on page 84)
- 2 whole dried apricots

Snack
- ½ ounce sunflower seeds and whole-wheat breadsticks (amount depending on size)

Dinner
- Eggplant Parmesan (recipe on page 229)
- ½ cup or more Italian green beans
- ½ to 1 cup fresh fruit salad

❧ SUNDAY

Breakfast
- Grapefruit broiled with a sprinkling of brown sugar
- 1 scrambled egg topped with ½ ounce cheese
- 2 slices whole-grain toast

Lunch
- Ratatouille (recipe on page 124)
- White beans tossed with olive oil, fresh lemon juice, and fresh or dried basil

Snack
- 1 ounce low-fat cheese on whole-grain crackers

Dinner
- French Cassoulet (recipe on page 186)
- Green salad and Olive Oil Vinaigrette (recipe on page 84)
- Homemade custard made with low-fat or nonfat milk and topped with berries

Resources

For more information on the Mediterranean diet, landscape, and lifestyle, take a look at these books and web sites.

🍞 BOOKS

The American Heart Association, *The New American Heart Association Cookbook: Twenty-fifth Anniversary Edition*. New York: Times Books, 1999.

Barrenechea, T., and Goodbody, M. *The Basque Table: Passionate Home Cooking from One of Europe's Great Regional Cuisines*. Harvard Common Press, 1998.

Boyle, M., and Zyla, G. *Personal Nutrition, Third Edition*. Minneapolis: West Publishing Company, 1996.

Gollman, B., and Pierce, K. *The Phytopia Cookbook: A World of Plant-Centered Cuisine*. Dallas: Phytopia, Inc., 1999.

Jenkins, N. H. *Flavors of Tuscany: Traditional Recipes from the Tuscan Countryside*. New York: Broadway Books, 1998.

Jenkins, N. H. *The Mediterranean Diet Cookbook: A Delicious Alternative for Lifelong Health*. New York: Bantam Books, 1994.

Jodice, M., and Matvejevic, P., *Mediterranean*. New York: Aperture, 1996.

Keys, A. B. *How to Eat Well and Stay Well the Mediterranean Way*.

Lovatt-Smith, L. *Mediterranean Living*. New York: Whitney Library of Design, 1998.

Mahan, K., and Escott-Stump, S. *Krause's Food, Nutrition, & Diet Therapy*. Philadelphia: W. B. Saunders Company 9th edition. 1996.

Ornish, D. *Program for Reversing Heart Disease, the Only System Scientifically Proven to Reverse Heart Disease without Drugs or Surgery*. New York: Ivy Books, 1996.

Pawlak, L. *A Perfect 10: Phyto "New-trients" against Cancers*. Berkely, CA: Biomed General Corp, 1998.

Pennington, J. *Bowes & Church's Food Values of Portions Commonly Used*. Philadelphia: Lippincott, 17th edition, 1998.

Rogers, J., ed. *Prevention's Quick and Healthy Low-Fat Cooking: Featuring Cuisines from the Mediterranean*. Rodale Press: 1994.

Romaine, D. and DeWitt, D. E. *The Complete Idiot's Guide to a Happy, Healthy Heart*. New York: Alpha/Macmillan USA, 1998.

Rosso, J. *Fresh Start: Great low-fat recipes, day-by-day menus—the savvy way to cook, eat, and live!* New York: Crown Publishers, 1996.

Rothfeld, G., and LeVert, S. *Folic Acid and the Amazing B Vitamins*. New York: Berkley Books, 2000.

St. Paul's Greek Orthodox Cathedral, (Ed)., *The Complete Book of Greek Cooking: The Recipe Club of St. Paul's Orthodox Cathedral* New York: HarperPerennial Library, 1991.

Schlesinger, S., and Earnest, B. *The Low-Cholesterol Olive Oil Cookbook: More Than 200 Recipes*. Villard Books, 1996.

Simopoulos, A. P. and Robinson, J. *The Omega Diet: The Lifesaving Nutritional Program Based on the Diet of the Island of Crete*. New York: HarperCollins, 1999.

Uvezian, S. *Recipes and Remembrances from an Eastern Mediterranean Kitchen: A Culinary Journey Through Syria, Lebanon, and Jordan*. Texas: University of Texas Press, 1999.

Weir, J. *From Tapas to Meze: First Courses from the Mediterranean Shores of Spain, France, Italy, Greece, Turkey, the Middle East, and North Africa*. New York: Crown Publishers, 1994.

Wells, P. Trattoria: *Healthy, Simple, Robust Fare Inspired by the Small Family Restaurants of Italy*. New York: William Morrow and Co., 1993.

Wolfert, P. *The Cooking of the Eastern Mediterranean: 215 Healthy, Vibrant, and Inspired Recipes*. New York: HarperCollins, 1994.

Wolfert, P. *Couscous and Other Good Foods from Morocco*. New York: HarperCollins, 1987.

Wolfert, P. *Mediterranean Grains and Greens: A Book of Savory, Sun-Drenched Recipes*. New York: HarperCollins, 1998.

Wolfert, P. *Mostly Mediterranean: More Than 200 Recipes from France, Spain, Greece, Morocco, and Sicily.* New York: Penguin USA, 1996.

Woodward, Sarah. *Classic Mediterranean Cookbook.* New York: Dorling Kindersley, 1995.

Wright, Clifford A. *A Mediterranean Feast: The Story of the Birth of the Celebrated Cuisines of the Mediterranean from the Merchants of Venice to the Barbary Corsairs.* New York: William Morrow & Co., 1999.

✆ WEB SITES

American Dietetic Association: *http://www.eatright.org/*

American Heart Association: *http://www.americanheart.org/*

American Journal of Clinical Nutrition: *http://www.ajcn.org/*

Cucina italiana.com, "The virtual home of Italian cuisine and the Mediterranean Diet": *http://www.cucinaitaliana.com/index.shtml*

DotPharmacy's "Life of the Med": *http://www.dotpharmacy.com/upmed.html*

Dr. Andrew Weil's Self-Healing (contains newsletter subscription information): *http://www.drweilselfhealing.com/*

Oldways Preservation and Exchange Trust: *http://www.oldwayspt.org/*

Tufts University Health and Nutrition Letter (includes subscription information): *http://healthletter.tufts.edu/*

Tufts University Nutrition Navigator (reviews nutrition-related web sites): *http://navigator.tufts.edu/*

U.S. Food and Drug Administration, "Internet FDA": *http://www.fda.gov/*

Index

Recipes denoted by *italic* page references